CitiusTech

D0619563

Dear folks,

As healthcare technology continues at an accelerated pace, internet and digitization will be key in driving the next wave of healthcare advancements. Breakthrough innovations and adoption of smart phones, wearables, IoT, etc., over the past few years have created enormous potential for care givers to extend their reach and deliver personalized care. Yet, sucessfully integrating these emerging opportunities with enterprise healthcare applications to deliver value to all stakeholders in an effective and secure manner remains a challenge.

The Internet of Healthy Things is an insightful book that captures critical aspects of digital healthcare with real-world instances. Packed with practical tips and strategies, the book highlights exploding opportunities that a connected health landscape can offer to the industry. We hope you enjoy reading it!

As a specialist provider of healthcare technology solutions, CitiusTech has had the opportunity to work with leading providers, payers and life sciences companies to support them in their digitial transformation initiatives.

We look forward to collaborating with you to accelerate innovation in healthcare and make a meaningful impact on human life.

Sincerely Yours,

Rizwan Koita
CEO, CitiusTech

THE INTERNET OF HEALTHY THINGS

THE INTERNET OF HEALTHY THINGS

Joseph C. Kvedar MD

Carol Colman and Gina Cella

Partners Connected Health

Partners Connected Health
25 New Chardon Street, 3rd Floor, Suite 300
Boston, MA 02114

Printed in the United States of America
Partners HealthCare Connected Health

First Printing, 2015

ISBN: 0692534571
ISBN-13: 9780692534571

www.theinternetofhealthythings.com

Contents

Acknowledgments

One of the reasons I rise each day at 5 a.m., travel happily to work and put in an average of 60 hours per week is that I learn each day. In a sense, each person I talk to is a teacher and I owe all of them a debt of gratitude. The lessons conveyed in this book come from a 20-year span of my career. During that time there have been countless meetings, conversations and insights, indeed from hundreds of teachers. I can't possibly acknowledge all of them, but I want to thank a few.

This book represents a true collaboration. The ideas and insights communicated are like thread and the resulting tapestry a unique working arrangement between my coauthors, Carol Colman and Gina Cella, and me. Their contributions can't be emphasized enough.

My mother and father provided me with a grounding in truth and honesty, as well as an appreciation for the value of learning and education—remarkable for two individuals whose most advanced education was high school. My brother, Tony, always encouraging and a stalwart supporter, though eight years my senior, was always at my side (if virtually) during my development.

My wife, Vicki, deserves tremendous credit for being the backbone of our family while I pursued my dreams. Our children, Derek, Julie and Megan, have always been supportive and encouraging, despite their desire to have more of their dad's attention than they individually got.

Professionally, the team surrounding me has done amazing work to turn my dreams into reality. All of the insights detailed in this book are a direct result of their work and the learning that comes from trial and error in the real world. In 20 years, there have been many high performers on the team. Most recently, the amazing combination of Kamal Jethwani, Susan Lane and Nancy Lugn has moved the execution of our vision to a new level. My assistant, Carola Roeder, who has managed my multifaceted professional life with great patience, professionalism and precision, deserves special mention. Countless individuals I come into contact with offer praise to Carola and, like all good assistants, she toils in the background, mostly unnoticed.

I have been blessed to have many wise and thoughtful mentors and supporters over my clinical career. Howard Baden took me into the Harvard system with no experience and minimal credentials. Tom Fitzpatrick offered me the dermatology residency that arguably changed my career, as it opened the door for my faculty appointment at Harvard Medical School, an enormous gift and opportunity for anyone.

John Parrish "assigned" me my first project in telemedicine and gave me years of seasoned advice afterward. Likewise, Jim Thrall had the vision for the Telemedicine Center at Massachusetts General Hospital, in 1994, to which I was appointed director, once again with little in the way of credentials or experience.

John Glaser offered me the opportunity to build a team. He was a unique healthcare CIO in that he shared my vision for time and place independent care and provided many years of executive cover when the concept was fledgling.

Four generations of Partners' CEOs have overseen our work, each providing his own unique brand of support: Sam Thier, Jim Mongan, Gary Gottlieb and, currently, David Torchiana. For the past year and a half, I've had the pleasure of working under Gregg Meyer, who has provided an enormous wealth of support and inspiration to our Partners Connected Health team.

In the early days, Marcia Reissig, currently CEO of Sutter VNA & Hospice, was an incredibly valuable collaborator. Marcia had a vision for how connected health could move the homecare industry forward that was well ahead of its time.

I've also been fortunate to have many outside advisors over the years. No matter how experienced you get, you never cease needing counsel and guidance. Jay Sanders, who was among the earliest pioneers in the field, has been a tremendous role model and guide. Likewise, Jack Connors, a civic leader of immense proportion in Boston, has always found the time to guide me, make connections and help me move the vision forward.

Many thanks as well to Dr. Harry Leider, who gave generously of his time not only to be interviewed, but to write the forward for this book.

It was enormously gratifying, when I reached out to a host of leaders in the field, asking them for their time to be interviewed for the book, that so many people generously gave of their time and wisdom. These individuals were interviewed and are quoted in the text: Dr. Neil Evans, co-director, Connected Health, Veterans Health Administration; Sean Duffy, CEO, Omada Health; Dr. Anand Iyer, chief data science officer, WellDoc; Bill Geary, general partner, Flare Capital Partners; Andy Palmer, co-founder, Tamr and Koa Labs; Dr. Noel Harvey, vice president, Research and Development, BD Technologies; Rob Havasy, vice president, Personal Connected Health Alliance and executive director, Continua; Brian McGoff, vice president, Yorn Health; Deven McGraw, deputy director for Health Information Privacy, U.S. Department of Health & Human Services, Office for Civil Rights; Dr. John Moore, co-founder and CEO Twine Health; Dr. Steve Ommen, associate dean, Center for Connected Care, Mayo Clinic; Paul Puopolo, vice president, Business Innovation and Development, Highmark; Karan Singh, co-founder, Ginger. io; Rick Valencia, senior vice president and general manager, Qualcomm Life, Inc.; Dr. Nick van Goor, head of Data Science, Honeywell Connected Homes.

In addition, Tim Hale, Kamal Jethwani, Susan Lane and Meghan Searl from our Partners Connected Health team were also interviewed and quoted.

The following individuals also gave of their time and offered wisdom that helped shape the book's content: Ariel Garten, co-founder and CEO, InteraXon; Dr. Mark Boguski, founder and chief medical officer, Precision Medicine Network, Inc.; Dr. George Church, professor of genetics, Harvard Medical School and director of PersonalGenomes.org.; Amy Cueva, founder and chief experience officer, Mad*Pow; Carl Dvorak, president, Epic; Dr. Frank Moss, serial entrepreneur, former director of the MIT Media Lab and co-founder and chairman, Twine Health; Dr. Deborah Rozman, president and co-CEO, HeartMath.

Last, but not least, a big thanks to our friends at Egg Design Partners for their work on the cover design for this book.

Foreword
by Harry L. Leider, MD, MBA

I've dedicated my career to improving the health of large populations with common conditions like diabetes, heart disease, obesity and asthma. I've pursued this goal as a leader within medical groups, health plans, companies focused on improving "population health" and now as chief medical officer of Walgreens. So when Joe Kvedar asked me to write the foreword to *The Internet of Healthy Things*, I was honored. You see, Joe and I share the same passion for improving the health of millions of people who want to get fit, lose weight, quit smoking, live independently as they age and better control chronic conditions like diabetes and heart disease. *This important book clearly explains how new smart devices and Internet-based technologies make it possible for healthcare providers and patients to work together to improve health in ways that are powerful and previously unimaginable.*

That's exactly the approach we're taking at Walgreens. In reality, we are building our own Internet of Healthy Things. We connect our pharmacists and nurse practitioners with consumers and their smart devices (smartphones, wearables, scales, glucometers, to name just a few) and now with physicians. We provide consumers with access to their own health data and reward them for taking steps to maintain and improve their health via our Walgreens app. (Joe lends his perspective to our work in Chapter 6, "Some Healthy Disruption.")

Like Joe, I remember the days when healthcare wasn't so "connected." I began this journey about 20 years ago and, prior to joining Walgreens, I focused on patients with a condition called heart failure. People with heart failure typically have a weak heart muscle due to a severe heart attack, alcohol abuse or as a result of a rare viral infection. The weakened heart causes blood to "back-up" into blood vessels in the lungs and legs. If the condition is uncontrolled, it causes swelling of the legs, progressive shortness of breath, frequent ER visits and hospitalizations, and can lead to death.

Back then, we often supported patients with severe heart failure by having a nurse call them every week to see if they were consistently taking critical medications to make it easier for the heart to pump blood. We also checked to make sure they were following a low-salt diet to reduce excess fluid buildup. The nurse asked patients to report their "morning weight," since an increase in body weight over a week or two predicts worsening heart failure and an impending hospitalization. If a patient's weight increased rapidly, the nurse would contact the patient's physician and have existing medications adjusted or new ones prescribed to reduce the fluid buildup —and often avert a medical emergency.

This approach works very well, and typically hospitalizations are reduced by 50%. Unfortunately, this model of providing patient support is very expensive. This is because each nurse can only support a "panel" of 75 patients, since the nurse must initiate many phone calls each day to gather information and intervene when necessary. While this model is financially viable for heart failure, it is not economically feasible for most chronic conditions where hospitalizations are less frequent and serious exacerbations of disease (diabetes, hypertension, high cholesterol, for example) occur over many years.

Fast forward 10 years. I am serving as an executive in another company that supports patients with heart failure—but uses new "connected health" technologies. We provide our patients with a "remote monitoring" system that consists of a special scale that they step on every morning before eating. The scale also has a pedestal and a touch screen that enables patients to answer simple preprogrammed questions such as "Are you more short of breath today?" Each morning the patient's weight and answers are transmitted over a standard telephone line through an Internet server to a computer that provides our nurses with an automatic alert whenever a patient rapidly gains weight or has worsening symptoms that suggest an impending crisis. Nurses review this data each day and proactively call only the highest risk patients and, when appropriate, alert their physicians.

This "management by exception" approach enabled our nurses to effectively manage over 300 patients simultaneously and simplified the lives of these patients, as they only had to weigh themselves each day. This was a compelling experience for me that demonstrated the power of smart devices and internet-based technology to transform healthcare.

No one has done more to power the creation of new models of healthcare delivery than Joe Kvedar and his colleagues at Partners HealthCare in Boston. Over the past two decades, they have relentlessly evaluated, developed and implemented innovative technologies to improve healthcare delivery and outcomes. Healthcare leaders throughout the world look to Joe and Partners Connected Health to better understand how emerging healthcare technologies can connect patients, healthcare providers and caregivers while empowering patients to take more responsibility for their health.

Early in *The Internet of Healthy Things*, Joe summarizes his mission as a pioneer in this exciting space: *Our job is to imagine the future—and then invent it. We ask ourselves, "What are the connected health devices and applications that our clinicians will be using five to 10 years from now?" and "What should we be doing right now to prepare for that future?"*

The future that Joe is speaking about is, in many ways, already here. We are facing a "perfect storm" of major forces driving the creation and adoption of new connected healthcare devices and technologies. These include a shortage of primary care physicians; the rise of healthcare consumerism; a migration to "pay-for-performance" models that compensate doctors and hospitals for improving quality of care; and the aging of our population. In a clear and compelling manner, Joe explains why these forces are triggering an unprecedented flood of capital into companies developing these technologies and how these trends are fueling the transformation of healthcare and the creation of the Internet of *Healthy* Things.

These forces are also driving the development of thousands of apps, devices, wearables, sensors and Internet-based tools that have uncertain value. In early 2015, I attended the Consumer Electronics Show in Las Vegas and one pavilion, the size of a football field, was filled with kiosks and booths promoting hundreds of different wearable devices. Almost all of them tracked the same things: Steps taken, miles walked, calories burned, hours slept and so on. Yet there was virtually no data presented on how successful these devices are in enabling users to get fit, lose weight or sleep better. Similarly, at the time of this publication, there are over 1,500 apps available to help people with diabetes better manage their condition—but again there is very sparse data on the value and impact of these tools.

Joe's book contains a wealth of real world examples of new "nodes" of innovation being built within the Internet of Healthy Things. These examples, and his insights, based on decades of experience, will help you better understand how and where real value is being created. This book also explores how new technologies must empower consumers to change behaviors to become healthier and to manage their chronic conditions. This connection is at the core of value creation—as data, technology and connectivity will not improve health unless they enable us to change our behaviors, or work more effectively with our healthcare providers and caregivers.

At Walgreens, I have the unique opportunity to work with other leaders within this iconic company to extend our incredible "brick-and-mortar" platform—with over 8,000 pharmacies, 25,000 pharmacists and 400 retail health clinics—into the digital space while offering additional convenient and high-quality services. We've done this in a variety of ways that are highly consistent with the principles laid out in this book.

We started with a Pharmacy Chat function that enables consumers to obtain instant information and advice from our pharmacists anytime and anywhere. We then created a widely popular program called *Balance Rewards for healthy choices.*® Participants earn our Balance Rewards points for taking small steps to improve their health, like logging steps, weight and blood pressure, or making important changes toward quitting smoking. These points are an incentive toward changing behavior, as they can be redeemed for a set dollar value toward the purchase of many Walgreen's products. We also enable participants to log their data and sync this data with their Balance Rewards account using a wide range of connected devices and apps, such as Fitbit and other wearables, connected scales, compatible glucometers and blood pressure cuffs.

Balance Rewards for healthy choices is probably the largest connected health platform in the world with more than 800,000 participants and over 400,000 connected devices and apps. At the time this book was published, participants had set over 1.5 million health goals and collectively walked over 73 million miles! While it is still too early to determine the total impact of this program, participants who log their weight lose an average of 3.3 pounds. They are also significantly more consistent in taking their medications for diabetes and high blood pressure. We have enhanced this program, in partnership with WebMD, by offering a range of "digital health advising" tools that enable users to set specific goals and receive useful advice on their smartphones, tablets or computers.

In addition, Walgreens now offers, in some states, an affordable telemedicine service with our partner MDLIVE. For many common conditions, our customers can schedule a telemedicine appointment with a board certified physician and have this "virtual video visit" at work, at home or wherever and whenever it is convenient.

These programs and other pharmacy and health support services are all integrated within a user-friendly experience in our award-winning Walgreens app.

The emerging phenomenon that Joe has so appropriately named the Internet of *Healthy* Things is thrilling and it is transforming healthcare across the world. That's why Joe Kvedar's *The Internet of Healthy Things* is a "must-read" book for anyone interested in innovation, technology and the future of our most valuable commodity—our health.

Introduction

Making the Connection

Today, at Partners HealthCare, it's commonplace for high-risk patients to track their blood pressure, blood glucose and weight at home and send that data wirelessly to their electronic medical records. It is also routine for doctors to capture images with their smartphones and forward them through the cloud to be reviewed by other doctors halfway around the world. Our 1.5 million patients—from the tech savvy digital natives to their octogenarian grandparents—are video-chatting with family members using tablets and smartphones and health tracking devices in increasing numbers. Wearables are all the rage and a big part of their value is the potential to improve health. Computing is now wireless and can be held in the palm of your hand. Furthermore, across the healthcare spectrum, hundreds of thousands of patients are being seen "virtually" via telehealth and tens of millions are downloading health apps.

Given where we are today, it's hard to imagine that just two decades ago, what we now call mHealth, digital health or connected health simply didn't exist. This book not only marks the twentieth anniversary of Partners HealthCare Connected Health, but the invention of a radically new way to deliver healthcare and inspire wellness. Through these past two decades, we have learned, grown, succeeded and failed. We have technologies available that were never even dreamed of just 10 years ago. And, importantly, we have a convergence of market dynamics that make connected health solutions a prime driver in changing healthcare delivery.

Connected health is mainstreaming in a rapid way, but as I talk to investors, entrepreneurs and business leaders, they are at a loss for what to do with this exploding opportunity. The space feels chaotic and they worry about healthcare—the complex, long sales cycles, the liability concerns, overregulation and the like. This book takes the lessons we've learned over the past 20 years and brings them all into focus, providing guidance on what investments, business strategies and technology considerations are necessary to achieve order (and profit) from the chaos.

Having been fortunate enough to enter this field from the ground floor, I'm proud to be among some of the earliest pioneers who helped invent it. However, when I attended medical school at the University of Vermont, doing something like this was the farthest thing from my mind. My training is in dermatology and I came to Boston after medical school in 1983, destined for an internship at Boston University Medical Center. A year later, by a somewhat circuitous route, I found myself working as a research fellow in a dermatology lab at Massachusetts General Hospital (MGH). That turned into a residency in dermatology and, in what seemed like the blink of an eye, I was junior faculty, working on skin differentiation funded by an early phase NIH grant. By 1993, however, this effort was in peril and I went to my chief, John Parrish, MD, to talk about other career options. The next several years were a blur as Dr. Parrish provided me with ample opportunity to try various career paths while remaining in academia.

This was around the time that large academic centers—like Partners—were first beginning to feel the impact of managed care and the restrictions that it placed upon providers. Specifically, a new insurance tool called *capitation*, which forced individual doctors to bear full risk for their patients, was being implemented in California and Massachusetts. My colleagues were up in arms as you might expect. Yet I was a bit disappointed by their response to the call to be more efficient, recognizing that the current way of doing business was incompatible with the new managed care mandates. In the back of my mind I had been thinking, "How can we attack this thing called capitation and still maintain high-quality care?" We didn't know the answer to the question, but we understood that we had to explore different options.

Back in the research lab, Dr. Parrish, always the visionary, wanted me to investigate whether a series of digital images could be of good enough quality to allow a dermatologist to render a diagnosis without ever physically examining the patient. This was pretty radical thinking. Rightly or wrongly, all physicians—but especially dermatologists—are trained to place a great deal of emphasis on the physical examination. The notion that an accurate diagnosis could be made remotely by a physician who had never even laid eyes on the patient bordered on medical heresy.

I was working on several experiments at the time, but this was the first that used a digital camera, in this case a one-megapixel resolution camera the size of a shoebox that cost a whopping $12,000! Using the camera, I photographed scores of common skin conditions from dermatology patients. I then uploaded the images to a computer in my lab, along with patient histories. Since this was before web browsers and I had no way of sending these images to another computer, I invited a colleague into the lab to analyze the pictures.

Much to my astonishment, my colleague sat down at the computer and quickly breezed through the images. Within two hours, he was able to offer a diagnosis for more than 20 cases—*almost twice as fast as in an office setting with the exact same degree of accuracy.* This was a life-changing epiphany. I realized that by removing the barrier requiring patient and doctor to be in the same place at the same time, it opened up all kinds of opportunities to create value and improve access, quality and efficiency. I was dazzled by this vision and began to pursue it with the zeal of a blind man seeing for the first time.

The rest is mostly a typical entrepreneurial story. In 1994, Massachusetts General Hospital, buoyed by the influence of Dr. Parrish and the chair of radiology, James Thrall, MD, formed a telemedicine center. I convinced them to bring me on as director and got a small budget and two half-time employees.

Although we had a great vision for future applications and for research, we were grounded by a specific business need: the collection of clinical materials from international clients so our MGH clinicians could remotely render a second opinion on these cases. Ironically, we did this with the most rudimentary technology (fax machines and occasional digitized x-rays). It was important, early on, to have a business need that was grounded. It solidified executive support while we got our act together and figured out how we were going to create the future.

It is worth mentioning that, at that time, traditional funding agencies (the National Institutes of Health, foundations and so on) had no interest in this area. We were largely viewed as the lunatic fringe. Luckily, some local executives shared our vision.

In 1994, Massachusetts General Hospital and Brigham and Women's Hospital joined forces to create the Partners HealthCare System. The inaugural chief information officer was John Glaser, PhD, and in the spring of 1995 he sought me out, asking if I'd join his team. He offered a significant increase in resources (the staff count of the group grew to six, increasing by 600%!). This was an important milestone, as a staff of six is enough to really start to get some things done. We also joined forces with a team of folks who were working on videoconferencing technology. We called ourselves Partners Telemedicine.

During the latter part of the 1990s, we worked to perfect the process of conducting remote second opinions all over the world. The value proposition was to increase access to the knowledge base of our outstanding Harvard Medical School–affiliated specialists. We also dabbled in other areas such as tele-education, which used videoconferencing as an administrative tool within our provider network, and the store-and-forward teledermatology program that got me interested in the first place. In addition, we worked to move our programs, when possible, onto the Internet.

You can just imagine how rough this phase was—none of the technologies were reliable, and they were all costly. We managed to land some international contracts and a proof of concept grant or two in order to survive some lean years. In 2001, we took our second opinion program online, creating Partners Online Specialty Consultations (POSC), which to this day continues to offer Internet-based second opinions to patients and healthcare providers all over the world.

Another contributing factor to our growth was Medicare's decision to pay for home care services using a model called prospective payment. The then-CEO of our Partners Home Care group, Marcia Reissig, RN, MS, was farsighted, recognizing the need to use technology as a tool to improve the reach of her home care nurses. This was critical for us, because it was the first instance when a business leader saw telehealth as an opportunity to increase efficiency. Together with Marcia and her team, we created our congestive heart failure (CHF) telemonitoring program, now called Connected Cardiac Care.

Today, patients are given a blood pressure cuff and weight scale, along with a small tabletop touchscreen, and are asked to upload their vital signs daily. These data are monitored by telemonitoring nurses at Partners HealthCare at Home. If a patient does not upload his or her data or a person's vitals are outside established clinical parameters, a nurse calls the patient immediately. The results have been gratifying. We've kept thousands of patients healthy in their homes and out of the emergency room.

This program, too, was ahead of its time and had its share of naysayers. Several cardiologists predicted that it would never work and many of the home care nurses worried that this new technology would drive a wedge between them and their patients. It took several years to ramp up, but we proved these concerns to be ill-founded. Patients actually do better on this program and feel more connected and better cared for. The Connected Cardiac Care program is now offered as standard of care to those CHF patients in our system who are at high risk for readmission to the hospital.

It was in 2004 that the chairman of the Partners board of directors, Jack Connors, became interested in home care for the elderly. This, in turn, piqued the interest of our then-CEO, Jim Mongan, MD. Jim formed a committee to explore opportunities for care in the home and I was asked to join.

In the fall of 2005, as a result of this committee work, our budget was more than doubled. Based on my assertion that the next important application of the technology would be caring for patients with chronic illness in the home, we set out to take the learning from our success with congestive heart failure patients and apply it to other illnesses, such as diabetes and hypertension.

Shortly thereafter, during a presentation to the Partners board, Jack Connors remarked that he felt the term "telehealth" was too limiting. At the time, most folks were disenchanted with traditional telehealth, citing adoption barriers including lack of reimbursement, challenges with interstate licensure and concerns about liability.

With his comment fresh in my mind, we started using the term connected health to embody this new way of thinking about telehealth, focusing on the value proposition of improved efficiency rather than on the more traditional access-based value proposition.

In January 2007, we rebranded our group, becoming the Center for Connected Health. This was one of the best decisions we ever made because it gave us something fresh to talk about. The industry responded well to this new term; it is widely used today.

We then set out to create what we now call our "Connect" programs, which allow us to monitor patients with hypertension and diabetes in the home. We also recognized the need to build a single technology platform that would enable us to collect patient-generated data and aggregate it in one data-base, so clinicians and patients would have a common view. In 2012, we were the first U.S. medical center to enable patient-generated data from a personal health device to be displayed in both our electronic health record and our patient portal.

Over several years, we worked with various home-monitoring technologies and learned a number of critical lessons. Collecting objective data from patients is important; device-generated readings are much better (more accurate) than self-reported readings. We discovered that when these programs are offered in a clinical setting, it's important for clinicians to participate. In fact, we have shown many times that clinical outcomes vary positively with both patient engagement and clinician engagement (a number of patients dropped out of programs because they felt like no one in their doctor's office was paying attention to their data). We also learned that patient-generated data enable us to measure patient engagement in a refined way and, because we know engagement correlates with outcomes, we can more finely segment our patient population using these tools.

Starting in 2008, we began to incorporate the use of mobile devices into our work. At that time, the smartphone was just gaining momentum, so we built our programs around text messaging in order to reach the largest segment of patients possible. Text messaging also enabled us to do something we were unable to do before—cross the digital divide to reach even the underserved who were avid cellphone users. Our initial foray into mobile health was developing a text messaging program for young, at-risk pregnant women and another for individuals enrolled in an opioid addiction treatment program. Both programs, offered in collaboration with one of our Partners health centers located in an underserved community outside of Boston, were successful as measured by increased interactivity from those patient groups with their doctors. This early work gave us insight into the power of in-the-moment messaging on a mobile platform and how that can increase patient engagement.

We've since developed, in collaboration with others, texting programs for smoking cessation and increasing activity. And as more and more patients have adopted smartphones (now in the range of 65% to 75% in our market) we are migrating these texting programs to apps and creating new ones, such as an app to help cancer patients better manage pain.

We are always looking for ways to bring our innovations to a large audience. In 2010, we founded and spun out a company, Healthrageous, to create connected health programs for health plans and employers using consumer/patient-generated data and automated coaching. I was a board observer and participated in the company's early strategy. It was a wild ride and I learned a tremendous amount. Healthrageous was acquired in 2013.

That same year, we also made our first foray into the consumer market, launching Wellocracy.com, a free source of impartial, easy-to-understand information on new personal "self-health" technologies like activity trackers, wearable devices and mobile apps. Our goal was to empower consumers to self-manage their health and wellness using these readily available technologies and devices.

As I will demonstrate in this book, connected health is also an ideal model for population-level care. When Partners became one of Medicare's Pioneer Accountable Care Organizations (ACOs), signing risk-bearing contracts with all of our Massachusetts-based payers, a decision was made to invest in population health. With this shift, my colleague Tim Ferris, MD, MPH, was appointed senior vice president of Population Health Management and was asked to create a population health strategy for Partners HealthCare. Building blocks such as team-based primary care (patient-centered medical home), population identification tools, predictive modeling and integrating mental health into primary care were put into place.

As a result, Tim's Population Health Management group has become an important internal customer of ours. Through their vision and collaboration, we've started the process of scaling programs such as Blood Pressure Connect and piloting other innovations such as electronic medication adherence tools. Tim's team has taken the lead on integrating virtual patient visits across the Partners system, starting with a well-run program at Massachusetts General Hospital.

Our work continues with an exemplary team of clinicians, technologists, strategists and innovators, focusing on validating new models of care delivery, integrating personal health technologies in clinical practice and addressing key challenges to decrease hospital readmissions, improve patient access to quality care and smooth the transition from the hospital to the home.

We took stock of our list of innovative projects and reasoned that we'd make a bigger difference if we could find collaborators to bring them to scale. For example, the CHF remote monitoring program we built with Partners HealthCare at Home is now run by their team of telemonitoring nurses. Susan Lane, RN, MSN, MBA, is passionate about our work and manages operations for our connected health programs, as well as doing consulting work on behalf of our clients.

The research team has grown under the leadership of Kamal Jethwani, MD, MPH. We are now focused on the goal of creating personalized, motivational, engaging messaging for each individual in order to help that person improve health and sustain behavior change. We have exciting collaborations ongoing with a number of firms including the Robert Wood Johnson Foundation, Daiichi-Sankyo and Samsung.

I must also recognize several important events in our history. First, in 2014, our team began reporting to the chief clinical officer at Partners, Gregg Meyer, MD. Gregg is a strong advocate for connected health and taught me what leadership really means. You'll find him quoted often in this book.

Another key development has been the enthusiasm of Dr. Tim Ferris, who recognized connected health as a tool for the next generation of population health. The leadership of these two gentlemen has made an enormous difference in moving the vision of connected health forward at Partners. This underscores the increasing role connected health will play at Partners' hospitals, including Brigham and Women's Hospital and Massachusetts General Hospital, as well as in today's accountable care environment.

We've come a very long way. When I started 20 years ago, I often felt like a lone wolf howling in the wilderness. What is remarkable to me is that the vision was so clear then and, despite many setbacks over the ensuing years, my team and I never wavered from the path forward to achieve it. On top of that, the business of healthcare is changing dramatically, with providers taking on risk for population-level care and consumers buying insurance on exchanges and paying a much larger part of their bills. And all of this medical information is available to patients on the Internet. The disease burden is changing, too, as we've largely conquered acute illnesses, such as infections, and must now deal with the ever-growing specter of lifestyle-related, chronic silent killers such as diabetes, hypertension, high cholesterol and obesity.

At Partners Connected Health we're just hitting our stride after 20 years. I may have been a bit ahead of my time when I started, but lucky for me I did not know it and did not let it deter me. Many of you in the field may have had similar experiences as well. When you have the kind of epiphany that I described earlier, the future becomes so clear, and the path so real, you feel the need to pursue it with zeal but also with the requisite patience required as the rest of the world catches on.

In terms of connected health, the world is indeed catching up. There are so many innovations in this vibrant field, I would never be able to cover everything in one book. Rather I have chosen a number of examples of companies doing work that I find innovative and inspiring. The flip side to this cauldron of innovation is enough chaos to make many companies tentative about dipping a toe in the water. This book is also meant to help them find a path.

We need all of you to work furiously at the challenge at hand. Healthcare delivery needs to change, becoming more efficient, more patient-centric. As

I'll discuss, this is a multifaceted challenge with many opportunities for success. My wish is that each of you takes something from this book that will enable you to take a risk, but do so with greater confidence.

—Joe Kvedar, MD, vice president,
Connected Health, Partners HealthCare

1

20/20 Foresight

"**G**ood morning, Joe. Today's date is October 30, 2020. The sun is shining and it's a great day to be outdoors."

I am awakened by a voice text from Sam, my Virtual Health Coach, assigned to me by my employer, Partners HealthCare, as part of our Great Health/Great Life initiative. Based on my preferences and personality type, Sam is a cross between a no-nonsense drill sergeant, personal trainer and occasional psychologist. I weigh myself, quickly shower, dress and go downstairs for breakfast.

As I open my iPad to review the morning news, I see my personal health dashboard as the splash screen. (This is part of the same program that brings me Sam, and by enrolling I reduced my healthcare premium by 20%.) I take a minute to review my vital statistics, which include my weight, blood pressure, sleep quality, activity level, cholesterol level and medication adherence. It also reminds me of my "heart age," an assessment of my heart health based on my biometrics and lifestyle data. Because of my family history and lipid profile, I'm supposed to take a statin drug every evening to lower my cholesterol. But I have to admit that, some days, I forget to take my medication without a reminder. The dashboard notes that I remembered to do it last night.

Sam pops up on the screen and says, "Joe, your blood pressure and cholesterol are fine, but your sleep deficit is now up to three hours for the week, you've put on two pounds since last month and your activity level is falling short of your goal by 25%. You'll have to get more sleep and exercise if you're going to achieve your goal of fitting into your size 40/34 tuxedo by March for your daughter Julie's wedding. Only 140 more days to go!"

Sam's right. It's been a rough week, packed with meetings that made it difficult to fit in enough active minutes, and late nights that have cut into my sleep. Both are necessary to shed those extra few pounds that I put on over the last couple of months.

Sam offers this suggestion: "Joe, if you park your car in the Arch Street garage about 10 blocks away from your office today, you can walk an extra mile, or an additional 4,000 steps based on your gait. But that means you'll have to leave within 15 minutes so that you can still make your 9:30 meeting."

I soon find myself creeping along in traffic, my usual half-hour commute slowed down by an accident. Sam interrupts NPR's *Morning Edition* to inform me that my heart rate has increased (monitored by sensors embedded in my steering wheel) and I am showing signs of excessive stress. He suggests that I take a few deep breaths and then gives me some good news: The accident has been cleared and traffic is moving, which means that I still have time to fit in the extra walk Sam suggested.

By the time I get to the office, I am invigorated by the mile walk from the more distant garage and feel calm and refreshed. But I find myself stuck in a meeting that lasts until noon. As the meeting is winding down, my watch vibrates with an alert: "You've been inactive for two hours. A 15-minute walk now will extend the likelihood that you'll be able to attend your oldest grand-child's college graduation."

I take a quick walk around the block, then return for my usual lunch of vegetables, hummus and fruit. But today I am tempted to top it off with a cookie. As I head out of the building, my watch buzzes with a message, "I'm guessing you're walking toward Pace's Bakery to get one of their big chocolate chip cookies. If you have this snack now, it will only set you back further in your goal of fitting into size 34 waist pants. Why not use those extra calories to have a glass of red wine with dinner tonight, which is also better for your heart."

I pass on the cookie and take another brisk walk around the block before heading back to the office. When I return to the building, I turn toward the elevator but then remember that I promised Sam that I would always try to take the stairs and walk up the three flights.

Right before I leave work, I receive a text from Sam, "Joe, have you thought about taking up swimming again? I have a coupon from the Boston Sports Club two blocks from your office offering a six-month membership at half price. On top of that incentive, there are five other people in your online social network considering this opportunity, and I see three time slots each week when you could meet at least one of them for a swim. You don't have to make up your mind right now, just think it over."

Seconds later, I get a text from Julie, "Dad, I think swimming is a great idea for you. Thanks for skipping the cookie! You'll look great in your tux!"

That evening, I eat a healthy dinner of vegetarian tacos and salad, and reward myself with a glass of Alban Syrah. After dinner, while I'm reviewing emails, I open the refrigerator and reach for a postprandial bit of chocolate. As I'm doing so, a message flashes on the refrigerator door, "Joe, one serving of chocolate is around 180 calories. Given your dietary goals, a cup of chamomile tea is a better choice." A picture of Julie flashes on the screen and I make myself a cup of tea instead.

At the end of the evening, I receive a text from my physician's team. "Joe, all in all, you're doing pretty well (we know that Sam can be tough on you). We think the suggestion of swimming is a good one and agree you can use more sleep. Please spend some time over the next few days contemplating which you want to work on first. If you try to do both, your history suggests you will fail at both, but if you focus on one, your history predicts you'll succeed. After you commit to one or the other, we can set some goals and monitor your progress. Have a good night's sleep!"

I look at the clock and see it's nearly 10 p.m. The bedroom lights begin to fade and the room is filled with soft, relaxing music. Time to hit the hay so I don't fall further behind on my sleep deficit.

2

Seeing Around Corners

When people ask me to describe our work at Partners HealthCare Connected Health, I tell them what I tell my team: Our job is to imagine the future—and then invent it. We ask ourselves, "What are the connected health devices and applications that our clinicians will be using five to 10 years from now?" and "What should we be doing *right now* to prepare for that future?" In reality, our task is to see around corners and anticipate what the world will be like in the next decade and decades to come. I confess that my Virtual Health Coach, Sam, as described in Chapter 1, is still very much a figment of my imagination. It's my vision of what healthcare could—and *should*—be like.

When Partners established what was originally called Partners Telemedicine in 1995, the vision of an easy, intuitive healthcare system—which seamlessly intervenes with people just when they need it—would have been considered something to aspire to, but certainly not within the realm of possibility. Today, it's no longer out of reach. In fact, it is truly within striking distance. We now have the tools to help people manage their health and wellness in ways that would have been inconceivable just a few years ago. A case in point, when we changed our name to the Center for Connected Health in 2007—to better reflect the broad range of our work in telehealth, remote care and disease and lifestyle management programs—mobile health, or mHeath, didn't even exist.

My journey in connected health began well before the Internet, cloud computing, ubiquitous sensors, social networks, tablets, e-readers, mobile phones and apps became part of the fabric of our everyday lives. I didn't know with what, with whom or how we would be connecting to our patients. I did, however, recognize the need for technologies that could deliver health in a manner independent of time and place. And I knew that healthcare should be available to people in the context of their everyday lives and that implementing care in this manner would improve both quality and efficiency.

Today, everything and everyone is connected. According to a 2015 Pew Research report, two-thirds of Americans own a smartphone. And a phone is no longer just a phone: It's a miniature handheld computer—a truly smart phone—from which you can search, text, track your pregnancy, control your home thermostat and give yourself an at-home electrocardiogram (EKG). A workout shirt is no longer just a T-shirt: It can be transformed into a "wearable" biometric tool that can measure your heart rate, breathing rate and blood pressure, and transmit that data back to your smartphone. A pill is no longer just a pill: It's an "ingestible tracker" that can monitor medication adherence. And a watch is no longer just a watch: It's a fully connected device that can track your activity level, calories burned and stress levels, and dial up your doctor or pharmacist on command.

And this is just the beginning. Experts predict that by 2020, 26 billion everyday objects will be able to capture, receive and share data via a vast, interconnected global network linked together by inexpensive sensors, GPS and the cloud. Just around the corner, real-time biometric data will be automatically captured and used to learn more about the impact of lifestyle on disease and wellness, and ultimately change behavior for the better.

At Partners, we've coined a term to describe this phenomenon: The Internet of Healthy Things, or IoHT for short. There's no doubt that the emerging IoHT has vast implications for the healthcare industry, but it will equally impact those who are not in the business of healthcare. Soon, anything will be able to link up to the IoHT. It is now possible for virtually *anybody* and *any object*—furniture, exercise equipment, kitchen appliances, clothing, jewelry and even the family car—to be equipped with an inexpensive wireless radio and tap into the IoHT. Companies that can figure out how to harness this technology and incorporate it into their products or services will reap significant benefits for themselves and society.

A TREND LONG IN THE MAKING

It's a given that over time, healthcare will gradually move out of the doctor's office and hospital and become a continuous function in your life. When I was a kid, growing up in the sixties and seventies, we went to the hospital for everything. It *was* the information system. Of course, over the past few decades, that has changed. By the end of the twentieth century, you could get your surgery in an outpatient facility, a radiology exam in another geographically separate facility and your lab work drawn at still another facility. Your doctor, admittedly with some effort, was able to coordinate all of this care and get all of the records, mostly through a fax machine. And with the advent of the internet, your radiology exam from the suburban facility was likely read by a radiologist half-way around the world in Australia.

Fast forward to 2014 when, in that year alone according to the American Telemedicine Association, there were 800,000 virtual video visits between providers and patients. It is now common for patients hospitalized for congestive heart failure (CHF) to be monitored remotely during their recovery at home. You can see the trajectory and where we'll be in five, 10 or 20 years.

This book describes the phenomena driving this trend and the business opportunities that will arise from it.

The IoHT will play a crucial role in reinventing an archaic healthcare system that is now facing its greatest challenges ever. This transformational technology comes at a time when the healthcare system is undergoing tumultuous changes that will be felt by everyone: consumers, payers, providers and vendors.

The system that has long been disparaged by critics as "unsustainable," "bloated" and "inefficient" is now facing its day of reckoning:

- The shortage of healthcare providers is real, and growing, while the number of people seeking care is increasing.
- Changing market dynamics—the shift in *how* and *where* healthcare is delivered and paid for—will alter the role that consumers, payers and providers play in the healthcare system.

- New technology will level the playing field, enabling consumers to make knowledgeable decisions about their health on their own and also force them to assume greater responsibility for their actions.
- Providers, payers and vendors who cannot adapt to these new economic models will become obsolete.

But this game-changing opportunity has implications far beyond fixing our healthcare system. Every employer, the aging baby boomer generation, governments around the world, forward-thinking businesses and a more health-conscious consumer population all have skin in this game.

WHY NOW?

Until recently, wellness and preventive healthcare ventures were considered by most investors to be noble, if not quixotic, misadventures that lacked a long-term, sustainable business model. Whether or not an idea was funded often had little to do with its merits and everything to do with whether it was reimbursable by insurers. As a result, the focus has been on treating a patient once they developed diabetes or a heart condition rather than on keeping individuals healthy. We all know that wellness is the right thing to do, but we've struggled to find who will pay for it.

Unfortunately, conventional fee-for-service reimbursement models have discouraged preventive technologies and services that would keep people healthy and out of the hospital. They did, however, encourage providers to run up the highest possible charges everywhere along the supply chain—for endless and often unnecessary tests, avoidable hospital stays and wasted prescriptions, to name just a few. In most cases, this was done in the spirit of providing "the best possible care," but it has gotten us to a bad place. The United States has the dubious distinction of spending more money per person on healthcare than any other country on the planet, yet achieving modest health outcomes at best.

For the last 10 years at least, I've heard how the growth in healthcare expenditures is unsustainable. The fact is, spending one out of five dollars of our Gross Domestic Product (GDP) on health chokes off spending on other important initiatives. There is a real effort on the part of public and private payers to drive the cost of healthcare down—and this must be done without sacrificing quality. It's become obvious to even the most skeptical observers that keeping people well is a lot cheaper than paying for them when they get sick!

For all of these reasons (and more) healthcare is ripe for disruption. From a care delivery perspective, 60% of our costs are labor; our processes are not streamlined; there is little automation. For the most part, the consumers of our services put up with a terrible customer experience—an experience most would not tolerate from their bank, airline or favorite retailer.

Those involved with providing healthcare services are prone to significant waste without even realizing it. Healthcare reimbursement is governed by complex and Byzantine rules that take armies of employees to ensure insurance claims are being properly submitted and paid. We spend little effort keeping our citizens healthy, with most of our resources focused on fixing people once they are sick.

Recent events have dragged the *$3 trillion-a-year* healthcare industry into the twenty-first century, albeit sometimes kicking and screaming. The growing economic burden of chronic disease, the Affordable Care Act (ACA) of 2010 that mandates health insurance for all and reimbursement reform that rewards efficiency and *penalizes* bad outcomes have set the stage for a massive shakeup.

As part of this revolution, two important concepts have emerged: Payment reform and the changing relationship between the patient and the healthcare system. First, payment reform, which rewards providers for delivering high-performance quality care and improved clinical outcomes for large groups or populations of patients (people with diabetes, for example), is sweeping the land. In spring 2015, the Secretary of Health and Human Services went on record saying that by 2018, 50% of Medicare payments would be through risk-sharing arrangements with providers. Private insurers are following suit, with 40% of payments in 2014 being somehow value-based. *Simply put, there is a stampede away from volume-based reimbursement to value-based reimbursement.*

Two other insurance trends deserve mention here because of their direct impact on consumers. One is the movement toward high-deductible health plans, especially in the context of the health insurance exchanges (HIEs) implemented as a result of the Affordable Care Act. This combination has moved the cost of care squarely into the hands of Americans and the resulting transparency will contribute to lowering costs. The other is the formation of narrow network health plans. These plans cost the consumer less, but steer care toward a very narrow group of doctors, most often because of their historic track record of providing cost-effective care. Since provider payment drives so much of the economics of healthcare in the United States, understanding how these intersecting trends affect provider and patient behavior is crucial to business success.

The second concept, the changing relationship between the patient and the healthcare system, is really a seismic shift. For centuries, we were led to believe doctors were the saviors who could fix all that ails us. Individuals, who were not held responsible for developing lifestyle-related conditions such as hypertension, heart disease, diabetes and obesity, just needed to visit their healthcare provider to treat their health problems. Everything was viewed as an accident or bad luck. That's all changing, as we now have the tools to educate, motivate and monitor individuals—and reward them—for better self-managing their own health and wellness. We are taking the onus off providers and putting responsibility on the shoulders of the individual.

If the strategic levers are pulled just right, you could imagine a provider organization offering its patients a program to improve health while educating them, individually, on how that program would help them better manage their yearly health bill. In this scenario, the provider does well because it is proactively managing a patient population; patients do well because they see the direct impact on their deductible expenses and the health plan; and society at large does well because the overall cost of care goes down. Technology and connectivity play a major role in this coordination. What is happening more and more often today is that patients are avoiding care because they do not want to pay down deductibles. They wait until they are sick enough to use high-cost services such as the emergency room or the inpatient service. Clearly there is an opportunity in achieving better coordination.

"WELL"-NO LONGER A FOUR LETTER WORD

For the first time, there is a groundswell in demand for products and services that promote wellness and make it easier to manage chronic conditions outside of conventional medical settings. Connecting to the IoHT presents a huge opportunity for all sectors of business and society, especially newcomers to the space with fresh, creative ideas. At long last, public and private money is flowing to companies and services that help consumers be well, get well and stay well.

I've learned that when you want to get a glimpse of how a tumultuous business environment can lead to opportunity, you talk to seasoned, early stage investors. One of my favorites to listen to is Bill Geary, a general partner at Flare Capital Partners. Geary recently observed that basic market forces are now applicable in healthcare in ways they never were before. "Healthcare has been an industry where return-on-investment (ROI) was not in the lexicon. People didn't think about ROI in healthcare because if you had a better device, a better drug, an improved treatment, it almost didn't matter what it cost; you simply had to focus on how to get it reimbursed and have the health insurer cover it. Once they did that, then you tried to influence physician and caregiver behavior so they prescribed, used or implemented it. Now, all that has changed."

According to Geary, the vast potential for change for the better in healthcare is attracting a new generation of entrepreneurs eager to make their mark. "Healthcare was never cool," he says. "It's the last industry to really be so dramatically impacted by technology innovation and the advent of the consumer. Now it's attracting top talent from other disciplines to develop apps and business solutions, and it's exciting to be a part of these high-value transformative companies, which can totally change the cost and care-quality equation addressing one of the largest universal needs in our country."

WHO CAN PLAY?

It's not just the young and idealistic who are leaping into the health space: Companies like Apple, Google, Samsung, Microsoft, Philips, IBM, Intel and even the Ford Motor Company, to name just a few, are the superstars staking claim to the consumer health space.

Health probably isn't the first thing that comes to mind when you think of Samsung, yet this tech company's recent investment in biopharmaceuticals and biosimilars (generic versions of biologics) has analysts predicting that it will soon dominate the generic drug market. How? By adding health and wellness programs that lead to better compliance and, presumably, strong consumer loyalty. To wit, Partners HealthCare signed a groundbreaking partnership agreement earlier this year with Samsung to develop personalized digital and mobile solutions for health and wellness, including software development and a clinical research program designed to deliver tools to improve chronic disease management.

But it's not just tech giants like Samsung that are linking to the IoHT. In the summer of 2014, ball boys at the U.S. Open tennis tournament wore form-fitting Ralph Lauren polo shirts that measured heart rate, as well as breathing and stress levels (ball girls' shirts were still under development). The public was so taken with the concept that Ralph Lauren debuted its PoloTech shirt for men in August 2015. Powered by Montreal-based OM Signal, the shirt teams with an app to offer "live biometrics, adaptive workouts and more." Also keeping up with the trend is fashion designer Tory Burch, who created a jewelry line for Fitbit in 2014 that promises to "transform your tracker into a super chic accessory for work or weekend." Furthermore, sports apparel brand Under Armour's purchase of diet app MyFitnessPal (with its 45 million active users) and personal training app Endomondo in February 2015 could turn this sportswear icon into a wellness juggernaut. Even Victoria's Secret is now offering a sports bra with built-in electrodes that hook up to a heart rate monitor.

And it's not only the big brands who are leading the charge into health. The lower cost of starting an IT business, from inexpensive mobile app development to pay-as-you-go cloud computing, is opening the door to disruptive newcomers and their investors. According to Rock Health, a digital health accelerator, 2014 was a banner year for connected health startups. The $2.3 billion raised in just the first quarter was more than the entire amount raised in all of 2013. And, in the first half of 2015, digital health is showing no signs of slowing down, bringing in $2.1 billion in funding, just short of the 2014 numbers. Rock Health also notes that the average deal size in 2015 was over $15 million, exceeding 2014's $14.6 million mark.

CONNECTED HEALTH TAKES OFF
When Partners HealthCare first started developing technology-driven care delivery, the mobile health market was nonexistent. Today, the growth projections for this relatively new industry are staggering. In 2012, the global market for mobile health was valued at $1.95 billion. Experts now predict it will reach $49 billion by 2020, with about one-third of revenues coming from the United States. (The wearable device market alone is poised to hit nearly $23 billion in 2015 and is projected to exceed $173 billion by 2020, according to a 2015 Research and Markets report.)

But selling devices and apps is just a small piece of the connected health market. The data footprint created by people using them is a potential gold mine. Personal tracking data contains a treasure trove of information about how people live, work, play and even think, which sheds a great deal of light on their lifestyle, including their habits and preferences.

This information is an invaluable tool to marketers and advertisers who want to sell stuff to people. But it is also an incredible resource for businesses, insurers, healthcare providers and entrepreneurs—even government health ministries—who need to better understand what motivates the health consumer. And they're willing to pay big bucks to anyone who can find useful trends in the billions of data points collected every day. In 2014, an *MIT Technology Review Business Report* noted that, according to McKinsey & Company, there is a huge demand for platforms and services—*a business the consulting firm values at $350 billion to $400 billion annually*—that make this data both accessible and actionable to consumers.

THE RIGHT FEEDBACK

There are also roadblocks that need to be overcome. Physicians must be able to exchange patient data freely and securely among themselves. And patients must be able to share their personal health data with their providers. This is the challenge of interoperability—the ability of different devices to communicate seamlessly and securely. In today's world, if you have a CT scan or lab test performed at one medical facility on Monday and are admitted to a different hospital on Tuesday, your tests would probably have to be repeated because the treating provider can't access your results. With the growing adoption of electronic medical records (EMR) and improved interoperability, this should soon change for the better.

The other big challenge that remains—the Holy Grail of connected health—is packaging that data in a way that inspires and motivates individuals to make positive behavior changes and better manage their own health and wellness.

Wirelessly connected sensors enable an important design principle of connected health: feedback loops. Once you capture personal health data from these devices, the first important thing to do is to feed it back to the individual from whom it came. Feedback loops are great for establishing awareness and changing a person's mindset about health. But we have learned through the years that merely spitting data back at people will not achieve the desired behavior changes. It takes a lot more than simply showing people the error of their ways to trigger improvement. Individuals have to feel as if you really understand them, know what they're going through and can offer the right advice at the right moment.

Right now, if you were to ask me for a model of what I think the IoHT should be like, I would have to look outside of health to one of my favorite companies, Nest. Nest is best known for creating thermostats, lights and other home devices that can be controlled through its smartphone app. But Nest has a bigger vision, as described on its website: "This is about working behind the scenes to anticipate people's needs and make their lives easier." Nest does this by taking in data from various sources, integrating it, communicating with the cloud and creating a customized product or experience that is relevant to a person's life. For example, as you continue to use the Nest thermostat, it continues to learn about you and your preferences and adjusts room temperature accordingly. This is precisely the approach we need to take with healthcare technology.

People want to feel cared for as individuals. Nest products work because they learn about individuals and anticipate their needs. Google's plan for its automated assistant, Google Now, is for it to do the same. When these tools work, they create a powerful bond between the brand and its users. Those of us in the business of improving the health of our citizens need to do this—we need to care about you and anticipate your needs—and those businesses that get it right early stand to profit greatly as the system undergoes these fundamental changes.

Much of the work that we do at Partners Connected Health revolves around studying behavior and learning what makes each person tick. In that way, we can create programs and apps that resonate with each individual—and that *feel* authentic and personal—even though they may be delivered automatically through a device. Indeed, much of our work is devoted to finding the "just right" pitch perfect approach for each patient, based on his or her preferences and needs. In the chapters that follow, I will describe how we do our research, what we've learned from it and how it informs how we work with our patients.

NOT A SURE THING

There's no question that the IoHT will create new revenue streams for nontraditional health businesses, as well as exciting potential for cross-industry partnerships. It also has the potential to transform health and wellness, making it simpler, more convenient and more relevant to people as they go about their everyday lives. If the IoHT works, it will not only keep people healthier and happier, but it could save society hundreds of billions of dollars in healthcare costs.

But these optimistic predictions come with a caveat. Success in this space is not a sure thing—not even for companies that have a great track record selling to consumers.

That's because consumers have historically been resistant to the health message, a topic that I will explore more deeply later in this book. Let's not forget that half of all patients don't take their medications as prescribed, and only a rare few can maintain weight loss on their own or stick to an exercise regimen. My point is, although the shift in power (and responsibility) in healthcare is moving rapidly to the individual, it would be naive to believe that everyone is chomping at the bit to take charge of their health. This may be true for some—especially for patient activists and health bloggers—but those of us who work with patients every day see a different side of the story. We see individuals who are often ambivalent about taking responsibility for their health. They want to do what's best for themselves, but they are often thwarted by self-imposed barriers that must be overcome before they can move from good intentions to action.

It's true that millions of consumers are already using connected health devices, including popular health and fitness trackers like Fitbit, Striiv, Nike + FuelBand and Jawbone Up. It's also true, however, that the current market for wearables and apps is largely focused on the minority of primarily younger people who are self-motivated and passionate about health and fitness, the Quantified Selfers, or data "junkies," who live by the numbers.

There is a vast, untapped market for devices and programs aimed at the majority of people who are not fitness buffs or Quantified Selfers; people who may care about their health but who don't have the motivation or know-how to do what it takes to maintain it. In order to truly succeed at population health and to rein in the costs, we need to migrate that enthusiasm to caring for the "not so fit and fabulous" crowd. We need to focus our efforts on reaching the mere mortals who struggle with their weight, who very often have one or two chronic conditions that need to be managed, who are less likely to buy a tracker or download an app and, even if they do, probably won't use it for very long.

At the same time, we need to engage physicians and other medical personnel in the process. Too often a poorly designed technology is foisted upon providers without any thought about how it will fit into their workflow or to whether it's streamlining a process or actually adding another layer of complexity. That also means health-tech developers and innovators must understand the needs of those on the front lines. I devote Chapter 5, which I title "The New White Coat Anxiety," to this often overlooked problem.

Mobile health offers us many transformational opportunities. We can embed sensors in just about anything that collects data and stores it in the cloud. We can use smartphones and tablets, televisions and cars to engage individuals around health content. We can display health-related information at just the right moment, in just the right context. We can use cameras on our smartphones to capture relevant health information, a physical injury, or to get a visual record of food intake. We can send personalized texts in-the-moment with contextually relevant, motivating messages based on data collected from real life behavior.

We clearly have the technology—with advances being made every day—to empower individuals to conveniently and unobtrusively care about their health without doing much heavy lifting. In order to be successful in the widespread adoption of these technologies, however, we must get consumer engagement absolutely right and break down barriers within the healthcare system.

CONNECTING TO BUSINESS

Today, Partners Connected Health is in the vanguard of changing business models for healthcare delivery and integrating wellness into our everyday lives via the products we use every day. Our Connected Health team works with companies that are exploring how they will fit into this new world and, most important of all, learning how they can reach health consumers. In addition to creating our own technologies and systems, we provide a living laboratory, where companies can test out their new technologies, devices and platforms in a real-world setting, with actual healthcare providers and patients.

I am personally as passionate about mentoring as I am about connected health. Our mission at Partners is not just to create programs to serve our own providers and patients, but to lead innovation and advance healthcare delivery universally. Throughout my tenure, I have learned a great deal about what works in connected health—and what doesn't. I am sharing these insights because I would like to help people avoid the same mistakes that our company and others have made along the way.

As healthcare delivery moves to a value-based compensation paradigm, and with the attendant emphasis on population health, prevention and wellness, connected health offers an opportunity to radically change how we think about and manage health for the better. That can only be done if we have a successful and vibrant commercial sector.

As I say throughout this book, selling health is tough, and not just to patients and consumers, but to the folks on the front-lines—hospital administrators and providers. Although they may understand that they need better ways to manage patient populations, healthcare is not known for quick change. In order to talk to providers in a way that will make them listen, we must understand their mindset. Providers need to clearly see how a new technology will improve both their bottom line and the lives of their patients. Anything less these days just isn't going to cut it. Despite all the discussion about cost cutting and making healthcare sustainable, which are important, you will find that physicians are obsessed with giving their patients high-quality care.

That is a much harder task and for businesses to succeed in that endeavor, they need guidance. This book provides that guidance based on 20 years of experiments, trial and error, and successful implementations in order to enable businesses to fast-forward and "do well by doing good."

Through the years, I've had the opportunity to meet and work with other innovators in the connected health space, as well as investors, business accelerators, industry leaders, patients, patient advocates and caregivers. Throughout this book, I will look at the varied approaches taken by a wide range of companies and startups tackling different pieces of the health and wellness puzzle. My role here is to educate and inform; I am not endorsing any particular company or program, and there are many worthy companies that I have not been able to include.

GETTING IT RIGHT

If we get it right, many stand to gain. This has implications across all industries, for businesses large and small. For consumer goods and services companies, it translates into greater customer loyalty, product differentiation and potentially new markets. For big employers, it means helping to create a healthier, more motivated and productive workforce with fewer absences and lower healthcare costs. For healthcare providers and health-related companies, it means being able to survive in a tougher, more competitive environment, improve efficiencies and increase provider and patient satisfaction. For start-ups and entrepreneurs, it means starting off on the right foot, armed with the tools that are essential for optimal interaction with consumers.

As healthcare moves away from a volume-based model toward a value-based model in an effort to cut costs and improve outcomes, there will be winners and losers.

The winners:

- Companies that can take advantage of the shift of risk from the health plans to providers stand to profit.
- Companies that create smart systems to not only collect and display data—which is what everyone is doing—but to actually correlate data to create a very rich tapestry on which we can do analytics have huge opportunities. Right now, for example, my daily step count is displayed next to my blood pressure readings, displayed next to my weight, displayed next to my sleep quality. But no one is "connecting the dots" for the consumer, offering a simple message that shows how one piece of data impacts another. Making this information mean-ingful for people in the context of their lives is critical for consumer/patient engagement.
- Companies that know how to collect data from a range of sources and make sense out of it in a way that is useful for healthcare will profit. Analytics—machine learning—is in its very earliest stages. Right now, even the most sophisticated analytics companies fall seriously short of producing the kind of *hyperpersonalized* information healthcare providers require to fully understand individuals and create the tools to motivate and engage patients long term.

- Companies that can make technology *frictionless,* that is create devices and systems that make health improvement easy and seamless for consumers, will profit enormously. That's because many consumer products are too complicated and/or unreliable to be useful to the very consumers who may need them the most.
- Companies that enable the ecosystem described in Chapter 1 all have an opportunity for success in this new world.

Who might the losers be, then?

- Hospitals with their huge investment in fixed assets (buildings, CT scanners, laboratories, and so on) are at great risk. As more and more care moves into the network and we are increasingly rewarded for keeping patients out of the hospital and emergency room, hospitals must be nimble in their pursuit of alternative business opportunities.
- Those who supply to hospitals and rely on the old-school business model of fee-for-service are also at risk.
- Big Pharma that is resistant to change.

In the chapters that follow, I will provide a roadmap for businesses, big and small, old and new, as well as for health veterans and novices alike, on how to survive and thrive in the new connected health ecosystem.

• • •

THE MISMATCH

The current healthcare system—which is based on early twentieth-century needs—is a serious mismatch for the challenges we are confronting in the twenty-first century. Our healthcare system was designed to treat acute problems in an episodic fashion, which is precisely how physicians are trained to practice medicine—and how they are reimbursed for their efforts. That worked well when the biggest healthcare problems were injuries like broken limbs, infectious diseases, heart attacks or gallstones. It doesn't work well, however, with modern-day lifestyle-related epidemics like obesity and Type 2 diabetes, which are overwhelming the healthcare system.

Today half of all adults in the United States have one or more chronic health conditions and 25% of all American adults have two or more chronic conditions that must be properly managed or they can lead to more serious, potentially deadly complications. More than one-third of adults and 17% of youth are obese and another third are overweight—two risk factors for a long list of ailments, including diabetes, heart disease and many different types of cancer. Some 29.1 million people, or 9.3% of the U.S. population, have diabetes—a disease that was considered an oddity when I was a kid. And that's not the worst of it. The U.S. Centers for Disease Control (CDC) predicts that the incidence of diabetes may *triple* by 2050. If we don't get this under control, diabetes has the potential to break the bank. The total cost of diabetes was a whopping $247 billion in 2013, representing a 41% increase over the previous five years. Out of this figure, $176 billion was paid in direct medical costs, the remaining $69 billion in lost productivity. Considering the fact that 86 million people in the United States over the age of 20 are *prediabetic*, without the right kind of intervention, the tab for treating these soon-to-be-diabetic patients will be astronomical.

Type 2 diabetes, high blood pressure and obesity are directly related to an unhealthy lifestyle: poor diet, not enough activity, poor sleep habits and the like. These are not diseases that can be adequately managed with the standard once or twice a year visit to the doctor's office; they require sustained changes in lifestyle and behavior. And that requires vigilance on the part of both patients and their physician or other medical professionals.

The usual practice of writing a prescription for a drug, advising a patient to "lose weight and get more exercise," or expecting an individual to successfully follow a recommended diet plan just doesn't work. People need ongoing and consistent support from advisers or authority figures, like their healthcare provider, who not only emphasize accountability, but also help them stay on track and nudge them back if they lapse. The right text at the right time, a thoughtful email or televisit from a doctor or medical coach, or a phone call from a nurse monitoring personal health data recorded by the patient sitting at home can prevent a potential problem from spiraling into an expensive and potentially dangerous medical issue. Yet in terms of reimbursement, there is little incentive to track patients outside of a traditional medical setting. As long as we continue in the "business as usual" mode, the mismatch will continue and the problems will get worse.

3

The Big Shakeup

"We have to drive down the cost of healthcare. We now have tools like patient-generated data, health trackers and other types of personal health devices to help us increase medication adherence and get people to better manage their own health, which ultimately will head off costs in the future. There are a lot of startup opportunities here—there's millions to be made because there are billions to be saved."

—Rob Havasy, MS, vice president, Personal Connected Health Alliance and executive director, Continua

Recently, I was at a meeting with representatives from major healthcare organizations, including hospital and health plan administrators, and a big data multinational that consults to banks and financial service companies. The head analyst for this data giant explained how sophisticated methods of mining and interpreting data have enabled the company to identify customers who posed the greatest risk of defaulting on their loans through constant surveillance of customers' spending habits and other behaviors. There wasn't an empty seat in the house, which was amazing because a few years earlier, I doubt we could have drummed up enough interest to fill the first row.

The purpose of our meeting was to discuss whether the lessons learned in financial services are transferable to healthcare. It stands to reason that by mining data generated by health and medical trackers, as well as prescription renewals, social media interactions, restaurant habits and the like, it could be possible to create algorithms to predict which people were most likely to fall ill, even years before the first sign of failing health. More importantly, data analytics can help physicians and hospitals better identify high-risk, non-compliant patients who are most likely to end up back in the hospital, often multiple times, costing the system staggering amounts of money. There is also the opportunity to learn enough about each individual so that we can auto-matically message a person in a way that is highly personalized and effective at motivating that person to stay healthy.

The high attendance at this meeting was a reflection of the massive shake-up occurring in the U.S. healthcare system that has turned the tables on the conventional business model. In the traditional fee-for-service model that re-imburses each hospital visit, test and procedure, there is little incentive to re-duce hospitalizations or improve efficiencies. The 5% of patients who require the most medical intervention and who cost the most are also the most prof-itable. Under new payment models that penalize (rather than reward) what have been defined as "avoidable" hospital readmissions, the revenue model is flipped. Efficiency is rewarded as long as quality of care is maintained.

This approach is a radical departure from how we have paid for healthcare in the past and one that is having a transformative impact on the industry.

Healthcare has historically been a business driven by the efficiency of moving patients through brick-and-mortar facilities (a hospital or doctor's of-fice, for example) and performing as many reimbursable tests and procedures as possible. Payers and providers have been slow to catch up to the new mobile and digital health world, where we now communicate with tools that resem-ble FaceTime, Skype, texting and apps. For the most part, patient-provider communication, other than face-to-face, has not been reimbursed at all. This means that there is little contact between providers and patients between ap-pointments, and once patients leave the building, they are pretty much left to fend for themselves.

Patients who don't understand their postdischarge medication protocols are often overwhelmed by the demands of managing a tricky condition like congestive heart failure or Type 2 diabetes (which requires dosing their insulin correctly). Many may fall prey to "revolving door syndrome": They are readmitted to the hospital nearly as quickly as they were discharged. A 2013 report by the Robert Wood Johnson Foundation reported that one out of five Medicare recipients who check into a hospital is readmitted within 30 days at an annual cost of $26 billion, of which $17 billion is for "return trips that need not happen if patients get the right care."

It's been an expensive way to do business. In 1970, healthcare costs accounted for 7.2% of the GDP; by 1985, they exceeded 10% of the GDP. Today they consume 17% of the GDP, or $2.9 trillion annually. That adds up to *$9,255 per person* in the United States annually—three times the amount spent by other wealthy nations. By 2020, healthcare costs are predicted to rise to more than $4 trillion, accounting for 20% of the GDP.

And where does all that money go? Not necessarily to making us healthier. According to a 2012 study, "Eliminating Waste in US Healthcare," published in *The Journal of the American Medical Association* (*JAMA*), between 20% and 30% of total healthcare expenditure is wasteful. That's right, this means we're paying nearly a trillion dollars a year more than we actually should. "Waste" in the study is defined as overtesting and overtreatment, poor coordination and communication that may also result in redundancies in care and/or medical errors, excessively high margins for basic products and service, billing errors, and out-and-out fraud.

Given the runaway costs and high degree of waste, most other industries would have been forced to change their ways a long time ago, but healthcare isn't just any other industry. With the rare exception of the concierge practitioner who is paid directly by patients, most physicians and hospitals rely on third-party payers to pick up the tab. And for the most part, payers have. Through the years, there have been attempts to rein in costs by creating more hoops to jump through to get tests, treatments and procedures approved or, as in the case of some health maintenance organizations (HMOs), burdening providers with draconian contracts that simply didn't work. Despite it all, the basic fee-for-service system has remained intact.

That is, until now.

THE NEW REALITY

The convergence of several powerful economic, social and technological meg-atrends is creating upheaval in the healthcare system, overcoming the head-winds that have been resistant to change. Precisely at a time when greater numbers of Americans are becoming insured, it is estimated that there will be a shortage of close to 100,000 physicians needed to care for this influx of patients by 2025. Consider this additional sobering statistic: By 2020, 22.2% of the U.S. population will be over 60 years old, placing an even greater de-mand on the already strained healthcare system, both financially and in terms of human resources.

The demand for services is growing at such a rate that if we continue to in-sist on face-to-face interactions as the only way to deliver care, we simply won't be able to train providers fast enough. It's no secret that there aren't going to be enough doctors and nurses to treat all the people who need care. Keep in mind that we already have shortages in many specialties, with primary care doctors topping the list, and there are rural areas of the United States where doctors are scarce to begin with. Even if we could train more providers, this would likely drive up costs even further. Some 60% of our costs in healthcare are human resources—the last thing we need is more people on the payroll! When I visit my doctor, I routinely run the gauntlet of six clinical staffers be-fore I actually get in to see her. In contrast, when I check out at Home Depot, there is one employee for every six check-out stations. The only way we can fix this costs-run-amuck situation is to spread more patients/consumers across our limited provider population. And the only way to do that is with technol-ogy. *The companies that help our industry achieve this goal, without our patients feeling cheated or our doctors feeling overwhelmed, will profit handsomely.*

In an effort to cut costs—and improve outcomes—both public and private payers are rapidly pulling the plug on fee-for-service reimbursement. Instead, they are implementing a variety of value-based payments that take into ac-count other factors like patient progress, satisfaction levels and the ability of the provider to prevent hospital readmissions. It's finally sinking in that pay-ment reform and outcomes-based reimbursement are here to stay and that the old business model is on its way to extinction. The new reality of healthcare has created an urgent need for solutions that have the potential to reduce costs and boost efficiencies, improve outcomes and enhance the patient experience. There are huge opportunities for businesses that can help providers keep individuals healthier, happier and engaged, not just when that patient is sitting in the doctor's office, but during all those real-life moments in-between.

One friend of mine who sees this change every day is Rick Valencia, senior vice president and general manager of Qualcomm Life, Inc., a subsidiary of wireless technology giant Qualcomm Incorporated. According to Rick, "There's a big difference in the types of conversations that we're having right now as compared to even 2013. In the past, we were mostly talking to innovation groups who were 'kicking the tires' and the conversation was about how they *might* consider using digital technologies. The conversation has shifted from it being an interesting or novel idea to it being a requirement. Now, they're telling us that within five to 10 years they're not going to have *any* fee-for-service business. They've got to figure out how to first bridge the transition and then live in the new world." Qualcomm Life is focused on device connectivity, care coordination and data management to power connected chronic care, transitional care and connected therapy management solutions.

What is desperately needed—and this is where the IoHT can make a real difference—are tools to keep people healthy in the first place. According to Kamal Jethwani, MD, MPH, our senior director of Connected Health Innovation at Partners HealthCare, "In primary care, the biggest need is chronic disease management, managing patients in a preventive, holistic, lifestyle-oriented fashion. We call it a 'full person perspective' rather than a disease or medical perspective," he says. "And we need it across all diseases, including asthma, diabetes, heart failure and hypertension. Preventive medicine, which is ignored a lot, has great ROI if done correctly. *Preventing someone from becoming a patient with diabetes is so much cheaper to a health system than curing or treating that person after the fact.*"

A SYSTEM IN TRANSITION

Healthcare is currently straddling two worlds—the old and the new—sharply demarcated by different payment models and, perhaps more importantly, by different philosophical approaches to what the practice of medicine is all about. Although the fee-for-service world is waning, it still exists. Forty percent of commercial payments to doctors in 2014 were in value-based arrangements, but that means that over half were not.

Undoubtedly, some providers will be reluctant to give up the profitable fee-for-service model for the riskier pay-for-performance model, even if it offers financial rewards for success. This is not just a shift in how providers are paid, it also requires a major change in how patients are cared for and a move to managing health in a real-time, real-life environment. It changes the role of the provider, especially the physician, emphasizing a team approach over the more hierarchal one in which a doctor is at the top of the pyramid. Some applaud these changes, others are wary of them. (I go into more depth on this topic in Chapter 5.)

Love it or hate it, the momentum is clearly in favor of payment reform. The fact that an increasing number of providers are finding themselves in shared risk arrangements has sparked a greater interest in connected health. The only way providers can survive in this new reality is by assessing and understanding the risk they are taking on with their population of patients. Yet, that information is impossible to obtain by reading a few notes scribbled on a chart by a doctor or nurse once or twice a year, or accepting at face value what a patient has to say when you are sitting face-to-face.

The new tools like data analytics and health trackers can help a provider better understand what a patient does in real life and that patient's true health status, putting the provider in a better position to intervene in a timely manner, before a patient runs into trouble. Electronic medical records that aggregate information from different sources are also absolutely vital. These tools are not only cost effective, but lead to better medicine and better clinical outcomes.

The new economic realities of healthcare are not only impacting providers, they are changing the way payers are doing business. In order to manage care costs, they must establish a new relationship with their consumers. As Paul Puopolo, vice president of Business Innovation and Development at Highmark, one of the largest health insurers in the United States, asserts, "We know that our business has to change. You can't just sell insurance—you have to offer lifestyle solutions that offer value to the individual." Paul is a really sharp guy who has his finger on the pulse of all of these changes.

He continues, "The challenge with this change is you have to get your insured to understand that's what you are—you are not there just to pay the claim. You've got to know who your membership is on a much more detailed level and be able to connect with them at the right time and be relevant or they'll tune you out. That means that we have to think more like retailers. We need to understand each person and understand what his or her lifestyle is like because it impacts how that person makes health decisions. If you can understand who the person is, and anticipate or predict that person's needs, then you can integrate your solutions when the person is ready for them."

A NEW WAY TO DO BUSINESS

Healthcare reform has driven a wave of provider reimbursement reform that has turned the old revenue model on its head in several ways. As noted earlier, there is a movement away from paying doctors and hospitals for units of services toward a model where they are paid for quality and outcomes.

Under the Affordable Care Act there have been several reforms in Medicare reimbursement that have challenged the fee-for-service model. For example, groups of doctors, hospitals and other providers can form Accountable Care Organizations (ACOs), which, as defined by the Centers for Medicare & Medicaid Services (CMS), "come together voluntarily to give coordinated, high quality care to Medicare patients." An ACO must care for a minimum of 5,000 patients for at least three years. Under the law, providers earn bonuses if they keep their patients healthy and out of the hospital. Other types of reimbursement reform include bundled payments, where an episode of care is defined and the provider is paid a flat fee for treating the condition (orthopedic and cardiac surgical procedures are the most common starting point).

Partners HealthCare is a Pioneer ACO. In aggregate, we are responsible for some 500,000 lives and have risk-bearing contracts with the federal government and our three largest local payers. We are also self-insured for our 60,000 or so employees and their dependents.

Today, there are more than 400 ACO programs nationwide. Although some provider organizations have dropped out and the program has some flaws, from my perspective it's provided an economic context for providers to explore ways to integrate sensors, mobile devices and virtual visits into their care delivery and better manage patient populations as well.

Providers who work together under the umbrella of an ACO stand to benefit if they share information, avoid redundancy and perform only the tests and services that are essential. It's a team-based approach as opposed to the fee-for-service model in which each link on the healthcare chain operates independently, leading to quickly escalating costs.

In an ACO setting, you might think that there would be the temptation to scrimp on services. But, the flip side of the coin is that payment is reduced or denied if a patient fares poorly due to inadequate treatment. Under a sepa rate incentive program, penalties can be levied against providers if their patients are readmitted to the hospital for follow-up within 30 days of discharge due to any number of common conditions.

Those providers who did not take the threat of fines seriously learned the hard way that Medicare meant business. Last January, according to *Kaiser Health News*, the typical bonus of $213,000 earned by large hospitals in shared risk arrangements was wiped out by steep fines—the average penalty was $1.2 million. Smaller hospitals earned bonuses of $32,000, which were offset by penalties of $131,000. Ouch! Clearly, this is still a work in progress.

The other important dimension to ACOs is that Medicare defines your population. In other words, if any patient in your ACO receives care within your organization, you are, not surprisingly, responsible for the cost of that care. But if a patient chooses to seek care at a competing hospital or provider organization, you will also be on the hook for standard Medicare reimbursement rates. That means, you'll be contributing to their profit margin and taking away from your own! This creates serious interest in maintaining patient loyalty and satisfaction, a radical concept for healthcare. It is also likely to produce the consumer-centric healthcare system we've been hearing so much about the past few years

Critics contend that ACOs are little more than retreads of cost-saving programs like "capitation" implemented by HMOs in the 1990s. Doctors were paid a flat amount "per member per month" to take care of individuals who were members of a health plan. This system managed to alienate—infuriate is actually the better word—both physicians and patients. It also resulted in many lawsuits being filed by plan members contending they were hurt by the payment plan.

There are some significant differences between capitation of the 1990s and today's ACOs. First, it's true that having the person with fiduciary duty manage your health is a potential conflict of interest. ACOs, however, are different in that participants assume risk at a system-wide level, insulating doctors from direct risk. Second, back then doctors didn't have the level of control over outcomes that they do today, which enables them to work within such a tight budget: We didn't have the data systems necessary for success. Now, the IT tools available for managing population-based payments—from registries to data analytics to connected health—are breathtaking. We're using all of them at Partners and our goal is to transform healthcare delivery.

THE HURDLES

Our current payment models dictate that care is delivered when two people meet at the same location at the same time. Although technologies like home computers, mobile phones and home health hubs can be leveraged to monitor patients and offer much needed guidance, in real time, to avert emergencies, there has been no mechanism to pay for it. Payers typically don't reimburse nearly as well—or at all—for preventive care services, let alone for care performed virtually or outside of a hospital or doctor's office. If I spend an hour looking at various quality dashboards and sending messages to patients whose data fall outside of clinical parameters, there has been no way to be compensated for that.

Recently, the Centers for Medicare & Medicaid Services announced a new current procedural terminology (CPT) reimbursement code for chronic care management (CCM). What's important here is that the new payment code acknowledges the value of care management that is not face-to-face and that is delivered by nonphysician providers. While it does not specifically call out remote monitoring as a tool, remote monitoring is an ideal use case. We will now be able to engage with providers, particularly primary care physicians, who have modernized their practices using a team-based patient-centered medical home strategy. The CCM code also enables us to approach the market with a ROI-based business proposition rather than some of the hand waving we've employed in the past. It is still early going, but I predict this new code will bring a big lift to connected health as a tool for chronic illness management.

THE RISE OF THE HEALTHCARE CONSUMER

It's not just providers and payers who are being shaken up by transformational change in healthcare, however. Once relegated to a passive role in the system, consumers are now driving a lot of their own healthcare decisions.

Around 60% of working-age Americans—some 150 million people—are covered by employer plans. Under the Affordable Care Act, everyone who is not covered by Medicare, Medicaid or an employer must obtain health insurance on their own through state-run health insurance exchanges.

As noted earlier, one important achievement of the Affordable Care Act was the formation of these health insurance exchanges, which have put consumers front-and-center in making choices around healthcare coverage. This, combined with the movement toward high-deductible health plans and health savings accounts, is making individuals much more aware of what health services cost. Cost awareness and transparency are important factors in bringing costs under control. Buying insurance via exchanges will inevitably lead to more price sensitivity and clear the way for a number of connected health solutions.

The downside is that high-deductible plans—some costing as much as $6,000 a year—may discourage people from seeking care. *USA Today's* in-depth report, "Dilemma over Deductibles: Costs Crippling Middle Class," published in January 2015, raised concerns over the impact of high-deductible plans. Citing the fact that the average deductible more than doubled in eight years, from $584 to $1,217 for individual coverage, the article states, "Coverage long considered the gold standard of health insurance now often requires workers to pay so much out-of-pocket that many feel they must skip doctor visits, put off medical procedures, avoid filling prescriptions and ration pills—much as the uninsured have done."

It's true that, for the first time, many consumers are feeling the pain of higher healthcare costs. Obviously, excessively high deductibles are not in a consumer's best interest and certainly not what the health law intended. The upside is that enlightened consumers are now shopping around for health as they would for any other commodity. They are asking about the cost of procedures ahead of time and comparison-shopping between one hospital and another. They are also noticing that a virtual visit with a doctor via a telehealth service could cost even less than their deductible for an office visit, and not require any travel.

As I mentioned in the last chapter, payers are introducing another new tool, called narrow networks, designed to control costs. These health plans offer affordable coverage as long as the consumer gets his or her care within a very restricted group of physicians and hospitals prescreened by the insurer and known to be low-cost providers. Most academic medical centers are excluded from these networks.

All of this cost-consciousness comes at a good time if you consider the availability of information about health systems and providers (not to mention diseases) that is available on the Internet. The era of democratized health information is upon us. For the past 10 years, it has altered the conversation between patients and providers regarding the details of their medical conditions. Finally, this dialogue is moving to the realm of cost. Patients are choosing not only on the basis of perceived quality, but also on cost-of-care as this information becomes available.

As Bill Geary of Flare Capital Partners explains, "Consumers now have a financial stake: They have financial responsibility, whether that's through paying an increased copay or having to choose between various insurance plans and employer programs that give them the economic incentive and power to be shoppers in the search for the best value. This has never happened before and fundamentally changes everything for all stakeholders."

THE WAY WE WANT TO PRACTICE MEDICINE

I've talked a great deal about the economic burden of healthcare because, frankly, that has been the underlying motivation for many of the reforms that we're living through now. It may surprise you to learn, however, that many of our doctors at Partners HealthCare (and elsewhere) are tired of the hamster's wheel of fee-for-service reimbursement and welcome the opportunity to rethink care delivery.

Gregg Meyer, MD, chief clinical officer at Partners HealthCare and a primary care physician, is one of them. "In the past, no good deed went unpunished. If I took care of a patient via email or counseled that patient over the phone or even had that patient take a 'selfie' of his throat and send it to me via text message so I could determine whether or not he had strep, that was a wonderful service that I provided and I did so willingly," Meyer says. "But the truth of the matter is, it actually hurt my practice and it hurt my colleagues because we didn't get paid for it. It was more convenient for my patient and a more enjoyable experience for me, but we lost. There was no mechanism for us to get paid for care other than meeting with patients face-to-face."

Meyer notes that even in the fee-for-service model, providers took on risk, but of a different kind. "When people were getting relatively uncoordinated care, there was an outside risk we weren't able to provide them with the level of care we were proud of and, oh by the way, it was a whole lot more difficult and less efficient to do. We weren't talking with each of the patient's doctors; we weren't able to move patients through seamlessly. There was always risk, but in that case, providers buried the risk in bad outcomes. Now we're taking a risk that's financial. It puts our performance on the line on the one hand, but also frees us up and allows us to practice medicine in the twenty-first century, the way we've always wanted to practice medicine. Now we have a mechanism to make it all work financially."

There will be winners and losers in this big shakeup. Those who benefited from high margins during the heyday of fee-for-service are doomed if they can't adapt. Among them are "Big Pharma," if it can't wean itself off the block-buster model, as well as the current crop of EMR vendors, if they can't reorient their systems to maximize revenue in the context of shared risk.

Providers who don't make themselves more accessible to patients will lose them to CVS MinuteClinics or to the acute care centers seemingly popping up on every street corner. In this regard, Walgreens is a triple threat: It not only operates walk-in healthcare clinics and offers digital health advisors and other online services, it is more than delighted to have consumers link trackers to their Balance Rewards program to earn points for everyday healthy activities. The company is well-primed for the IoHT.

But the biggest challenge will be for hospitals. Their success is built on caring for sick patients and using a series of capital-intensive fixed assets to do so. Over the past two decades, we've seen the death of the bookstore, the music store and the travel agent, to name a few businesses that have gone by the wayside. What will be the fate of the hospital as we move into the world of risk-based contracting and connected health?

CHANGE IS COMING: ARE YOU READY?

The changes taking place in healthcare delivery are dramatic and far-reaching and will impact everyone—providers, payers, consumers and vendors alike. In short:

- Provider reimbursement is changing from "pay-for-volume" to "pay-for-value." Our former CEO, Jim Mongan, MD, succinctly characterized the effect this will have on providers by saying, "All of our high-margin items become costs and all of our costs become opportunities for efficiency."
- Consumers are facing new insurance products that are at once more complex but give infinitely more choice. Most of them include some sort of high deductible or narrow network.
- Because of healthcare reform, the Centers for Medicare & Medicaid Services is rolling out a new approach to hospital and physician payment. This includes tools such as the aforementioned Accountable

Care Organizations, the readmissions penalties and the new code for reimbursing non-face-to-face care.

During the transition, we'll need to invest in new tools and models of care as we start to jettison some of our old ways. Firms are used to thinking, "If it's for medical purposes, we can charge lots of money and justify it by calling it medical grade," and providers simply raise their fees and pass the cost on to payers. This is one of the reasons we're spending $3 trillion on healthcare. New solutions have to be efficient and affordable. We healthcare providers are starting to treat our suppliers the same way Walmart does. They're a company well-known for pressuring suppliers to give them the lowest possible price because they command such a high volume of distribution. As providers take on risk, they will be much less friendly to these other segments, especially when it comes to high-priced new drugs and devices. We are already prescribing generics almost exclusively and looking for the lowest possible cost for devices.

Who stands to gain as we transition to this new model? *Simply put, companies that help to get us there in an efficient way.* The opportunity for companies that help us identify which patients may require our intervention is vast and far reaching. These include process redesign firms, data analytics and predictive modeling firms, as well as electronic medical records and documentation firms. To sum up:

- Anyone who can help us get critical information from patients without bringing them into the healthcare system could be a winner. The Walgreens partnership with Theranos, a consumer healthcare technology company, is a wonderful example of this: Individuals will be able to get lab tests done quickly and cheaply at the corner drugstore. Another example is the advent of retail clinics where people can go for a defined set of conditions that are easy to diagnose and treat algorithmically.
- Connectivity and mobility are paving the way for us to create true continuous, time and place independent care. Companies (like

Vidyo) that are developing tools that allow for virtual care, such as patient-to-provider communications tools or that are facilitating the collection of patient-generated health data (like Qualcomm Life), are on the right track.

- In the late 1990s, during the first Dot-Com boom, many companies succeeded and failed, but those who bet on infrastructure providers (Telecos, ISPs and of course FedEx and UPS) did well. The analogous companies in this healthcare migration will be electronic medical records providers and firms that help us deal with security and privacy concerns.
- The companies that offer providers an opportunity to extend their human resources across more patients (in primary care the vernacular for this is "increased panel size") will reap huge benefits as long as consumers do not feel cheated of their relationship with their doctors and health professionals do not feel overwhelmed with work. We learned these last two lessons during the first wave of capitation and managed care in the 1990s.

  And who stands to lose as we turn the healthcare system upside down?

- In the healthcare provider ecosystem, hospitals are at greatest risk. They have enormous investments in fixed costs (buildings, laboratories, radiology scanners), which will make it difficult for them to adapt quickly as care moves to a more distributed model.
- The pharmaceutical industry—for all kinds of reasons—is in a panic. When our delivery system began to experiment with risk-sharing several years ago, the first thing we did was more or less ban brand name drugs and focus almost exclusively on generics. We cut off access to pharmaceutical sales people. This is why you see all of the pharma industry talking about (and in some cases implementing) strategies they call "beyond the pill."
- The big medical device companies are at risk too. We're putting pressure on them to standardize and commoditize as well.

• • •

THE PARABLE OF RADIOLOGY

When I was a medical student, radiology was a highly desired profession. Individuals, often with analytic, visual minds, found this way of making a living quite suitable. They worked pretty standard shift hours and had a relatively stress-free life, insulated from the burden of direct patient care. After interpreting black and white images for eight or so hours a day, they went home to their families and, in the process, commanded salaries in the mid–six figures.

When I had my epiphany and entered the world of connected health, tele-radiology was already quite well established. Radiology departments, particularly at academic centers, were investing in systems that allowed all radiology to be captured and read digitally. I remember watching a radiologist sit at a screen and read films taken in Saudi Arabia, Massachusetts, and several other countries and U.S. states in succession, without knowledge or concern about where the images had come from. This was a glimpse of what time and place independent care would look like.

Coincidentally, Thomas Friedman's 2005 book, *The World Is Flat*, came out right about the time things changed for U.S.-based radiologists. You see, many of these physicians grew tired of taking calls at night in order to provide services to hospitals and emergency rooms that inevitably had a need for radiologists' services during off hours. Connected health allowed for a solution.

Radiology service providers, famously called nighthawk services, began cropping up. These companies hired U.S.-trained radiologists living in countries halfway across the world, but importantly, in countries where the cost of living was lower and the expected wages of the physicians were correspondingly lower. These companies happily agreed to read films from U.S.-based hospitals during off hours. When it was nighttime in Boston, it was midday in Australia, so why not? The difference in the charge for the read and the cost of labor overseas became margin for these firms.

You can guess the rest of the story. If you can read films cheaper in Australia at midday, then why not during the night too? During the last several years, radiology has become a commodity business with downward pressure on reimbursements. The next time you have an x-ray taken, it could be read by a (highly qualified but less expensive) doctor overseas.

Has quality suffered? Not measurably. Have patients noticed a lapse in service? There is no evidence that I am aware of.

Depending on your perspective, this is either a cautionary tale or a liberating one. It is exemplary of the type of disruption that healthcare services are ripe for.

4

The Hardest Sell

"Whatever the 'connected' health thing of the future turns out to be—whether it's an app or a watch or something else we haven't even dreamed up yet—the goal will be the same. The future of health is proactive, self-managed wellness. We want to put the onus back on the person. We're saying, 'It's your health and I'm no longer your babysitter.' The reality is, it was too expensive doing it the old way."

—KAMAL JETHWANI, MD, MPH, SENIOR DIRECTOR, CONNECTED HEALTH INNOVATION, PARTNERS HEALTHCARE

"You can't educate people to better health. You have to engage them and support them in learning it for themselves."

—JOHN MOORE, MD, PHD, CO-FOUNDER AND CEO, TWINE HEALTH

About five years ago, Partners HealthCare conducted a study to test a remote data transmission technology for patients to use at home. We asked 30 patients with high blood pressure being treated at Massachusetts General Hospital to take their blood pressure daily and upload the results to a database via the Internet, so that a nurse could monitor their condition. Half the patients were given a wireless blood pressure device that automatically uploaded their data. The other half were given small home monitoring device hubs with a modem-based data transfer device that required them to press a button—that's it, just press a button—once a day to upload their data. We had pretty good compliance from the group using the wireless technology, and for the first two days of the study, two patients using the modem-based data collection method took their blood pressure and pressed the button. But by day three, it was down to only one in the modem group. *After that, radio silence. Not a single patient pressed the button.*

Needless to say, we were very frustrated, if not baffled, by these results. If we couldn't get people to press a button once a day to improve their health, how were we ever going to get them to take their medication, watch what they eat, get more exercise and, in general, do what they needed to do to stay well?

The moral of this story is simple: Putting technology into people's hands is no guarantee that they'll use it. It takes a good deal more to inspire people to change deep-rooted behaviors, even if they understand their risk factors and sincerely want to turn their lives around. Studies like this one, as well as our work with thousands of other patients, have taught us that it isn't enough to simply design devices and software. We need to put just as much effort into trying to break the code of human behavior.

An interesting part of our job is finding ways to get people to "press the button" along with delivering the right tools to help them make positive and sustainable changes in their lives. In this regard, we've also had some extraordinary—and at times unexpected—successes. In one recent study involving people with diabetes, our behavior-change strategies worked better in normalizing blood sugar than a leading drug! In retrospect, we achieved success when we expanded our focus beyond device design to understanding the mindset of the health consumer. We asked ourselves, "What is it about health that makes it such a hard sell?" And we also asked the even more puzzling question, "Why are people so resistant to doing what's good for them?"

Getting to the heart of human behavior is perhaps the most challenging task confronting the healthcare system. A sizable chunk of our healthcare spend—some estimates are as high as 70% of overall healthcare costs—is due to chronic illnesses like Type 2 diabetes, heart disease and different forms of cancer, many of which can be linked to inactivity and poor eating habits. From a provider perspective, if we can't get patients to assume more responsibility for their lifestyle and health, we will never be able to survive in a system that expects us to take on greater risk and judges us on outcomes.

There's only so much we can do from the top down to keep people well. Eventually, if the healthcare system is going to be transformed into one that is both effective and sustainable, individuals are going to have to take charge of their own health. For some, this new approach may feel like "empowerment"; others may think we're just trying to pass the buck. But the new reality is there's no other way to reduce costs, keep people healthier and meet the needs of the growing numbers of individuals who need healthcare, notably the newly insured and the rapidly growing aging population.

Our politicians have not helped us on this one. They prefer to emphasize what they are giving constituents and tend to shy away from discussions of accountability or narrowing choices. The political narrative is almost always about universal insurance coverage. The logic goes something like this: If you are sick (and thus a victim), you deserve coverage and the government would like to help you with that. This is great for the slice of illness that is related to bad luck, accidents or faulty genetics. However, when we conflate that victim mentality to lifestyle-induced conditions such as Type 2 diabetes, obesity and the like, we excuse you from any accountability for your own destiny. As provider organizations take on financial risk for the cost of care for populations, there is growing frustration, especially among primary care providers, that there is no "pay for performance for patients," as one of my colleagues once mused.

"MUST HAVE" VS. "MUST DO"

Much of the discussion about the big shakeup in healthcare has centered on saving money for public and private payers. However, this is not a compelling argument for consumers, especially since many are not seeing cost savings. Instead, their out-of-pocket expenses are going up! If this shift in healthcare—placing more responsibility on individuals for their own health and wellness—is not done correctly, there will be a backlash. People will feel that they are paying more for less care.

But the reality is, if we get this right, we'll not only get a handle on costs, but we'll also actually be providing *better* care. I mention this because when it comes to healthcare, *quality matters more than quantity*, an important point that is often lost in the ongoing debates about the future of care delivery. As healthcare becomes more personalized, as technology enables us to monitor our patients in real time and provide the right intervention at just the right time, our patients will not need as many office visits, diagnostic tests or procedures. Individuals will be empowered and motivated to live healthier lifestyles and many acute-care challenges can be reduced or even eliminated. Ultimately, many ER visits and hospital stays will be averted. *In this case, less really is more.*

Admittedly, some forms of DIY health will be easier to sell to consumers than others. Below, I include three interesting examples in which the patient or consumer benefits from the convenience of in-home care and the health system benefits from improved cost-efficiency. How do we split up the cost? The accountability? You could argue that the health system should give these things away to patients because of the gains in population management and efficiency (that is what we currently do with home blood pressure monitoring). You could also argue that consumers will see value in the convenience and should pay. The adage that anything free has no value comes into play here. (Attempts in the last decade to remove copays for certain drugs have largely been abandoned because adherence to therapy did not improve.) Some people even argue that we should pay our patients to achieve better outcomes! The thinking is all over the map and there is no definitive research. In the near future, we'll be investigating a model where we subsidize the cost of these programs, but where the consumer has some skin in the game too. With high deductible plans, perhaps this will all start to make sense.

Example 1: If you have a child who is susceptible to ear infections, investing $79 in an Oto Home, an otoscope produced by CellScope, may be a no brainer, especially if you are a busy professional who values your time. This small device attaches to an iPhone and enables parents to take an image inside their child's ear from home and send it to a medical professional who can then quickly evaluate the image remotely. Using this simple tool, parents may be able to avoid a trip to the pediatrician, not to mention benefit by helping their child to feel better faster. We'd all agree value is created, but how the cost and accountabilities are split up is still controversial. When talking to patients, I've also heard the loud refrain, "Why doesn't my health plan cover that expense?"

Example 2: When easy-to-use home blood collection kits become mainstream—the ones that require only a tiny pinprick to get a sample—you'd think that many people would sign on. It's far easier to draw blood at home and send it to a designated laboratory for analysis than to make a special trip to a lab or doctor's office just for a blood test. With the at-home kit, if the results are normal, people could even be spared the need for an annual physical. All communication with the lab or physician could then be conducted through texts and emails, bypassing the face-to-face office visit.

Once again, this may sound like a valuable timesaving proposition to some, but others have said to us, in focus groups, "Please don't take my yearly visit with my doctor away. I enjoy my time with her." The annual physical is a social event for some. Does that justify the cost if we can do without it? My interpretation of that comment is that we need to do better with our in-home programs so people don't long for the annual trip to their MD.

Example 3: As smartphones and tablets become ubiquitous, you would think that many patients with hypertension would gladly use an iHealth or Withings wireless cuff to keep tabs on their blood pressure readings. These wireless devices send the data directly to providers, eliminating the need for patients to go to the doctor's office every six months—or even more often—to have their blood pressure taken. These simple personal health tools provide straightforward, easy to quantify, immediate benefits. However, each requires an investment on the part of the consumer, both in terms of dollars and in terms of technology set up. One must download an app, pair a device to a smartphone or tablet, and so on. Remember the story I told above of "pushing one button"? All of a sudden, that seems like a piece of cake.

The next level of DIY health is going to be an even more difficult sell. It's a much different story that's needed to convince individuals to make constructive lifestyle changes, like reducing sugar intake, walking more and sitting less, and getting more sleep. That's because the benefits derived from these kinds of positive behavior changes are long term—and the pleasures from the bad habits are immediate. And although trackers and other devices can help monitor progress, making a behavior change requires a concerted effort. It can be hard work and there are a lot of outside forces that can undermine a person's best efforts.

The IoHT can go a long way in helping to create a culture of health. It's hard to maintain "self-control" when you encounter fast food restaurants on every block, are faced with supermarket shelves stocked with processed foods of dubious nutritive value and are barraged by a constant stream of advertising for products that are bad for your health. But the right device or app can be a constant companion, a best friend or coach who steers you away from temptation and trouble, overriding the negative forces trying to undermine your willpower.

THE ENGAGEMENT GAP

The IoHT can achieve its potential only if consumers are receptive to it. But so far, adoption of health tech has been uneven. Beyond a few well-known success stories, mobile health technologies have been slow to gain traction, even among the most motivated people. There may be 165,000 health-related apps sold in 62 online stores, but the vast majority are never downloaded. Out of those apps that are downloaded, the vast majority are deserted within two weeks. Although one out of five people over the age of 18 owns an activity tracker, studies have shown that within six months, one-third stop using the tracker altogether. Market watchers predict that 1.7 billion people will download a mobile health app by 2017. . . but no one can say for sure how many will actually be put to use.

The once favorable "buzz" around fitness trackers may be dying down. An August 2015 report by Argus Insights, the Los Gatos, California research company that uses big data to track consumer sentiment, has reported a noticeable decline in consumer interest in the fitness wearables market for the first half of 2015. Why? As Argus Insights founder and CEO, John Feland, explained in the company's press release announcing the study, "Consumers expect their wearables to do more than simply count steps." Noting that consumers are showing more interest in smartwatches that can do more than collect data, Feland adds, "It is clear that as the Apple Watch, the Moto 360, and the LG Watch Urbane outperform fitness bands in the hearts of consumers, Fitbit and others in this category will need to add more to their offerings to keep consumers engaged and coming back for more."

I would argue that unless Apple Watch and other smartwatches and wearables show that they can provide real value to consumers in terms of helping them achieve their wellness goals in a meaningful way, they too will fall by the wayside.

The lack of "stickiness" for trackers and apps is similar to the low retention rates experienced by the diet and fitness industry. About 90% of dieters give up within a year's time and some two-thirds of people stop using a gym membership within a few months after buying it. Getting people to try something new is easy—getting people to keep doing it once the initial novelty wears off, well, that's the hard part.

These lackluster figures should give pause to anyone trying to gain a foothold in the IoHT. Just because you build it, and people come, doesn't mean that they're going to stay.

This could be a disaster for companies planning their business models around continued consumption, for example, by selling additional goods, accessories and services to enhance the consumer experience. It could also be the death knell for the mobile health industry. Like other consumer products, if people see that their friends and relatives who invested in health devices like trackers are not using them, the market will eventually fizzle.

This is even true for companies with a successful track record in marketing consumer goods. Just because a company has a knack for marketing smartphones, TVs, cars or electric toothbrushes doesn't guarantee that it's going to be good at selling health.

The one wild card in this disruption of healthcare has been and always will be consumers. It takes a great deal of effort to move a health consumer from thought to action. Health consumers are very different creatures from people in the market for a new car or who are shopping around for the latest high-definition TV. And so far, when it comes to adopting health technology, consumers have been pretty fickle.

Even very successful consumer companies have tried their hand at health and failed. In 2008, Google launched Google Health, a place for consumers to store their personal health records. But the Internet giant abandoned it three years later because few people were using it. Microsoft's HealthVault, another health data repository, is currently dying on the vine for lack of use. The fact that both of these companies, after failed attempts at capturing the health consumer, are reentering the connected health market is yet another example of how irresistible—and lucrative—corporate America views this space. Yet, the question remains, will these companies fare any better this time around? My answer is: They will face the same fate unless they come to understand the difference between selling *cool tech* and selling *health tech*.

First, launching any new consumer product is a challenge in a marketplace where about 80% of all new products are doomed to fail. Even good products that people need and use can end up badly. Second, selling health is even harder. Health is a sensitive, personal issue that taps into our deepest fears and insecurities.

THEY'RE NOT BUYING IT

The value proposition for personal health devices is markedly different than selling typical consumer goods and services. The operating assumption among technologists is that standard adoption models will apply to *every* product they bring to market. That is, tech savvy early adopters will lead the way and eventually different market segments will sign on until a product is mainstreamed. This adoption model is in keeping with Geoffrey A. Moore's book, *Crossing the Chasm: Marketing and Selling High-Tech Products to Mainstream Customers*, first published in 2001. His work is touted as "the bible for bringing cutting-edge products to progressively larger markets."

When it comes to adoption models, nearly every business school graduate has studied the late Everett Rogers's diffusion of innovation model, which divides the adoption cycle into four distinct phases: early adopters, early majority, late majority and laggards. Although Rogers's and Moore's models may be valid for irresistible technologies like big-screen TVs, smartphones and tablets, they haven't panned out in terms of health—there are still far too many laggards! Yet, for the most part, technology companies are relying on adoption models for their health-tech devices as if they were iPhones or some other cool tech gadget. This is proving to be a mistake.

Health tech doesn't generate that same kind of excitement and, let's face it, health devices are often associated with a lot of negative imagery, including illness, discomfort, advancing age and anxiety. There's a huge difference in how most consumers perceive cool-fun tech (like smartphones and tablets) and how they feel about health tech.

Most successful consumer app development is based on fulfilling a basic, almost brainstem, human need. Snapchat, Instagram, and Tinder, all wildly popular apps and/or online communities, are designed to do this in a very simple way. Whether it's sending a private (and disposable) text or photo, posting a picture or video, or finding Mr. or Ms. Right, the goal is clear and the benefits are instantaneous. The challenge in healthcare is that, although we may know what individuals must do to improve their health, it is rarely fun and the basic human need component isn't easily activated. What seems more compelling is the stuff of late night infomercials: magic pills and potions that allow you to eat all you want and do whatever you want and still stay slim, sexy and healthy. The desire for the quick fix makes building "sticky" health apps and devices much tougher than launching a messaging or photo-sharing app.

One of the biggest hurdles is that health tools and trackers make demands on people that other products don't. Most successful consumer products offer tangible if not immediate rewards. They make life easier in terms of helping you complete a task better or more quickly, or they provide instant gratification—they taste good or make you feel or look good (and the real blockbusters are the ones that do it all). As a rule, successful consumer products don't require a lot of work and self-reflection, and you don't have to wait 10 or 20 years to reap their full benefits.

In contrast, health devices almost always require some form of self-analysis followed by behavior change. The goal of health apps and devices is to nudge us into doing things that we don't normally want to do—like going for a walk when we'd rather be lying on the couch watching *Game of Thrones* or reaching for an apple instead of grabbing a cookie or taking a medication that we would just as soon avoid. The trick is making this healthy behavior stick, not just for a few days or weeks at a time, but for a lifetime. For most folks, the elusive promise of a healthier future is not enough of a reason to keep going.

It's worth mentioning here that most of the conditions we hope to modify (excess calorie intake, high blood pressure, high cholesterol and insulin resistance) are silent in their attack. Think about how different this conversation would be if high blood pressure were more like having a broken arm. There is little need for a smartphone app or device to remind you to favor your sprained ankle or to soothe your headache. This paradox of how we evolved heightens the challenge of engaging people in healthy behaviors. Unhealthy behaviors often have an immediate reward and some component of pleasure. Healthy behaviors usually have a long-term payoff, require extra effort and are not that much fun.

IGNORANCE IS BLISS

For many people, health technologies may reveal things about themselves that they'd rather not know. Ignorance really is bliss. If you have no idea that your blood sugar is edging up every year, you can still have your cake and eat it guilt free. But when you know that you're at risk for diabetes and are tracking your blood glucose levels, the dessert that you once loved quickly becomes a source of anxiety. To compound the problem, our brain is pulling us in a different—and potentially destructive—direction. As Meghan Searl, PhD, a neuropsychologist who worked for many years at Partners Connected Health, so aptly puts it, "The brain is wired for pleasure, wants instant gratification, prefers good news over bad and likes to hear information that validates preconceptions. But that's not what health is about."

One of the problems derailing the adoption of health tech is the fact that we have all underestimated consumer resistance to the health message. This was especially true for some of the innovators first entering this space. These companies based most of their assumptions on the experiences of early adopters who, as it turns out, are hardly representative of the general public. Early adopters tend to be either fitter and younger or more tech-oriented than the average consumer. The "I'd rather not know" philosophy shared by many is in direct contrast to the beliefs held by health technology's early adopters—individuals who didn't fear more information but actually embraced it. For example, fitness trackers were initially marketed to elite athletes and fitness buffs who used them to monitor and enhance performance. For the most part, these people don't have the self-control issues that plague us mere mortals. Foregoing dessert, getting up at dawn to maintain their six-pack abs and watching every morsel they put into their mouths is a means to an end. For these folks, the bigger goal supersedes the sacrifices.

Similarly, Quantified Self enthusiasts are genuinely excited about gathering biometrics and tracking every detail about how their bodies function. They revel in this kind of information—and the more the better. By and large, these "recreational" users of health tech are not representative of the 50% of all people over the age of 50 who have at least one chronic health condition and who could really benefit from health tracking.

When it comes to health, there are often self-imposed barriers and fears that need to be broken down before an individual will even be willing to listen to a health message, let alone act on one. Selling wellness takes a lot more than making someone aware of his or her actions by spitting their health data back at them and then hoping it's enough to instigate behavior change. Creating a path to positive, sustainable change requires a sophisticated understanding of each person as an individual and then finding the "hook" that catches and keeps that person's attention and loyalty.

The problem is, very few devices and platforms in the health space demonstrate a deep understanding of the mindset of the health consumer. Sure, these gadgets may have sleek designs and enough bells and whistles to pass the coolness test. *But what nearly all of these devices lack are the behavioral incentives required to maintain the user's interest.* In other words, most are simply automating, not innovating.

A 2013 study of 30 of the most popular weight loss apps published in the *American Journal of Preventive Medicine* found, according to study author

Sherry Pagoto, PhD, that "Strategies that often were missing are ones that help patients with adherence and motivation."

There's no question that it takes significantly more effort on the part of device designers to create platforms that maintain consumer interest and, more importantly, keep people focused on changing their behavior. If it were easy—if making lifestyle changes weren't such a struggle—we wouldn't need health-tech devices in the first place.

DEEP IN DENIAL

Most physicians know not to take everything a patient says at face value, nor do we expect that every patient will listen to us. The reality is, most of the time patients don't follow a doctor's orders, even if they say they do. Some 50% of all prescriptions don't get filled or taken correctly and 90% of advice such as "lose some weight" or "get more exercise" gets ignored. Another reality is that patients aren't usually honest with their doctors, often telling us what they think we want to hear as opposed to what they actually do. We call this the *social desirability bias.*

For example, as a dermatologist, I have spent a good deal of time advising patients to use sunscreen every day as a means of preventing skin cancer. I have seen my fair share of patients who swear up and down that they *always* use sunscreen. They're so convincing that I'd almost believe them except that their deep, golden glow is a dead giveaway of their hours of sun exposure without sunscreen. In contrast, I have found close to 100% adherence to sunscreen use among patients who have been diagnosed with skin cancer. I find this very frustrating because I know that many of these cancers might have been prevented by vigilant use of sunscreen from an early age. The problem is, it can take years for skin cancer to develop after excessive sun exposure and it can do its damage slowly, over time.

My point is, it's very difficult to get people to wrap their brains around a problem that seems so far down the road that it's dissociated from current behavior. Social scientists who study how and why people make decisions tell us that the human brain has difficulty grasping abstract notions. It's a throwback to the days when our primitive brain—the one that responded to imminent danger from saber-toothed tigers and the like—was essential for our survival. If we don't feel an immediate impact from our actions (touch fire, get burned; annoy saber-toothed tiger, get eaten; go out without clothes in the winter, freeze to death), we have difficulty making the connection between present actions and our future selves.

WAITING IN AMBUSH

Today's biggest health threats are "stealth diseases" that are symptomless and cause their harm silently, over time. These are conditions that can easily be ignored. High blood pressure is a great example of a stealth disease. Unless you make a habit of checking your blood pressure regularly, high blood pressure is virtually undetectable until it reaches acute crisis levels. (That's why it's called the *silent* killer.) The stroke or heart attack that occurs with no prior symptoms was probably years in the making. Type 2 diabetes, a virtual epidemic today, is another stealth disease. Normal blood sugar is around 100, but most people can tolerate a blood glucose level of 150 to 200 or even higher without experiencing any untoward symptoms. That's why so many cases of Type 2 diabetes go untreated until they trigger some other downstream problem, like nerve damage, kidney malfunction or blindness.

Furthermore, even people who may be self-aware in other areas of their lives may be surprisingly unrealistic when it comes to their health. Numerous studies have shown that people tend to inflate their healthy behaviors and downplay their unhealthy practices. One, led by Brian Wansink, PhD, director of Cornell University's Food and Brand Lab, shows that people routinely underestimate the number of calories they consume; the more food on their plate, the higher the disconnect between reality and perception. And a recent British study found a "huge gap" between overweight people's self-reported sugar consumption and the actual sugar content in their food. To make matters worse, people typically *overestimate* their levels of daily physical activity. In a society in which food is plentiful, most jobs are sedentary and many communities don't even have sidewalks for pedestrians, it's no wonder that two-thirds of the U.S. population is either overweight or obese!

A huge challenge is convincing individuals that they actually have a potentially serious medical condition when they are experiencing no symptoms. Amy Bilodeau, RPh, a clinical pharmacist at Brigham and Women's Hospital in Boston, often encounters patients who are referred to her because they have been diagnosed with hypertension—but they don't believe it. These patients claim their high reading at their annual checkup is due to the fact that they are nervous in front of the doctor or nurse and, therefore, they don't really have high blood pressure and certainly don't need to take actions to treat it. Simply sending these patients home with a bottle of pills is worthless because they won't take them. Instead, Bilodeau suggests that these skeptical patients participate in our Partners HealthCare home monitoring program, Blood Pressure Connect, so they can check their BP daily from the comfort of their own homes and see for themselves if it's really a problem. By regularly monitoring their blood pressure, they quickly learn that their high readings cannot be considered "white coat hypertension," but rather are a health concern that needs to be addressed. Once individuals are shown that they do, in fact, have high blood pressure, they are more compliant about making lifestyle changes or taking their medication. To be sure, this involves a bit more interaction than simply handing a patient a prescription, but if it spares the patient from having a heart attack or stroke down the road, it is well worth it.

EDUCATION ISN'T INSPIRATION

Wearing an activity tracker that monitors your daily activity level, calories burned, stress levels and other biometrics is helpful in terms of making people more aware of their behaviors. We may not be conscious of the damage our diet or lack of activity is inflicting on our bodies as it is happening, but we can be made aware of the behaviors that are driving us down this destructive road. Combined with appropriate motivational strategies, this awareness can be powerful in steering people in the right direction.

It's important to remember, however, that education is not inspiration. By that I mean giving someone an intellectual understanding of a problem doesn't necessarily mean that they're going to take action. Some 18% of Americans still smoke despite the widespread educational campaigns and grim warnings against it.

And here's the kicker: Even medical professionals don't follow doctor's orders. A survey of 2,975 health professionals published in *The Journal of the American Medical Association* found that 8% were current smokers; 2% among physicians and 25% among licensed practical nurses. Furthermore, a 2012 study led by Sara Bleich, PhD, of the Johns Hopkins Bloomberg School of Public Health, found that about half of primary care providers are overweight. Although the rate of overweight physicians and nurses is better than the national average for overweight people in general, it's still surprisingly high if you consider the well-known connection between poor body mass index (BMI) and other health problems.

If anyone should understand the risks of bad behavior and live a healthy lifestyle, it's a medical professional. But, we're human too, and when the waiting room is overloaded with patients, or we're exhausted from a 24-hour shift, we're just as likely to reach for the first available snack and skip exercise as the next person. Yes, health is a very hard sell.

A CULTURAL DIVIDE

Ironically, when it comes to health, the most difficult sell is often to those who need it the most. Tim Hale, PhD, associate director of User Centered Design at Partners Connected Health and a research scientist at Harvard Medical School, knows this well. Hale's research focuses on how new information and communication technologies (ICTs) are transforming existing models of healthcare and the emergence of "digital health lifestyles." He has studied the role technology plays within different socioeconomic groups and how this can impact health disparities. For one thing, affluent children tend to live in homes where there may be multiple computers or tablets, including right in their own bedrooms. Like their parents, these kids tend to use technology as a means of gathering information. Have a question? It's the most natural thing in the world to reach for your device for an answer. Kids who are raised in less affluent homes may have to go to a library to access a computer and probably don't get to spend the same amount of time exploring the online world.

Hale notes that this can translate into offline activities as well. "They take the practical approach of, 'What can I do very quickly to achieve my goals?' They don't develop the same skills in terms of comparing information from different resources," Hale says.

Over time, the digital gap is closing, not necessarily with home computers, which are falling out of favor, but with smartphones and tablets. We've found that more than 60% of our disadvantaged patients own a smartphone and I suspect that the number will keep growing. And, according to Pew Research Center, 50% of American adults have a tablet or e-reader. While we've seen growing numbers of people in our underserved communities using smartphones, we have not seen the same adoption of health trackers, nor do our underserved patients download as many fitness and health apps as do our patients with more financial resources.

According to Hale, even if you get technology into the hands of all people, there is still a disparity in how different socioeconomic groups use it. He explains, "People who are more disadvantaged tend to use their devices more for entertainment purposes, whereas people from other backgrounds tend to do more information-seeking, more educational-type activities online."

These differences are far-reaching. Hale adds that children tend to duplicate the behavior of their parents in many activities, but this is especially true for health. For example, people who grow up in economically challenged circumstances may have different attitudes toward food than people who are more financially stable. The person who fears hunger may equate quantity with value—the concept of a supersized meal at a bargain price may be very appealing. And the oft repeated advice, "Eat five to 10 servings of fruits and vegetables daily," may resonate with people who have access to greengrocers, farmers' markets and a bit more income to pay for higher-priced produce. But eating fresh fruits and vegetables every day may seem impossible to people with a lower income or to those who live in urban or rural "food deserts" that have none of these conveniences. For some, the nearest salad may be the one sold at a fast food franchise, and the challenge is to get them to order that instead of the fries.

I'm not mentioning these differences to stigmatize different communities. Rather, it's important to understand that a "one size fits all message" will not work. If we are to bridge the health gap between the affluent and the underserved, it's important to anticipate these differences and find ways to engage people that are meaningful to them.

CLOSING THE GAP

All this isn't to say that consumers don't want new ways to manage their health and wellness. In fact, people have indicated that they're willing to pay for help getting healthier. A Harris Interactive poll conducted in September 2014 by Wellocracy (a free online community we created at Partners HealthCare to engage consumers in using wearables, activity trackers and other personal connected health technologies) found that 27% of American adults had used wearable activity trackers and apps to manage their health within the past year. Of that group, more than 75% reported that they would gladly pay for personalized feedback from a doctor, fitness trainer, coach, nutritionist, nurse or dietitian. It's not that consumers are rejecting connected health—not at all. They just want it to be better, more relatable and about them.

There's no question that the businesses that create the platforms that actually *engage* individuals will be the winners in this space. The "engagement gap" between people and their health *has* to change. Chronic, preventable disease is not only weighing down world economies, but is destroying the quality of life for *billions* of people.

Engagement is tough. That's why it's the topic of the bulk of this book. Building engaging products is a challenge. Here are some pointers for success:

- Personalize as much as possible. Our goal is to message each individual in a way that resonates with that person. The more you can learn about an individual and the more you can contextualize the message you send, the better.

- Focus on what is relevant right now and fit your health message in alongside it. We've shown many times that if people get a message that is relevant to their life they'll read it and thank you. Chances are they won't remember the health message, but they will be engaging in the healthy behavior.
- No one has cracked the nut of sustainability. We need programs that engage people for long periods of time.

Healthy behavior *is* the hardest sell. But we have many successful individuals and companies that have gotten our attention in nonhealthcare settings. We must take lessons from them. This is a challenge we must conquer.

5

The New White Coat Anxiety

"In the mid-20th century, physicians were the pillars of any community. If you were smart and sincere and ambitious, at the top of your class, there was nothing nobler or more rewarding that you could aspire to become. Today medicine is just another profession, and doctors have become like everybody else: insecure, discontented and anxious about the future."

—SANDEEP JAUHAR, MD, DIRECTOR OF THE HEART FAILURE
PROGRAM AT THE LONG ISLAND JEWISH MEDICAL CENTER;
FROM "WHY DOCTORS ARE SICK OF THEIR PROFESSION,"
WALL STREET JOURNAL, AUGUST 29, 2014

"Their schedules are so packed, they haven't any time to breath. Asking a practitioner to add one more thing to her day is like trying to change the tires on a moving train—it's nearly impossible."

—SUSAN LANE, RN, MSN, MBA, SENIOR DIRECTOR,
CONNECTED HEALTH OPERATIONS, PARTNERS HEALTHCARE

It's safe to say that many of my physician brethren are unhappy with their lot. I understand that the mountains of paperwork, incomprehensible and often exasperating billing procedures and waiting rooms packed to the rafters can be quite maddening. That said, I personally believe that the positive aspects of being a physician far outweigh the negatives. To me it is a privilege to make a good living helping to relieve the suffering of others. Yet, I concede that there is a great deal of discontent among the ranks, some of it valid.

My point in writing this chapter is not to air the grievances of physicians to garner sympathy, but to give you a better picture of what the person on the other end of your sales pitch is thinking. If you're going to sell your "disruptive" innovation to this challenging group of professionals, you need to understand the mindset of today's physician. And yes, you will have to sell—and sell hard—to doctors to get any meaningful traction and a piece of that $3 trillion being spent on healthcare.

The reason this is crucial is that physicians universally have the ultimate say in how healthcare is delivered, at least in the industrialized world. On the delivery side, they are the decision makers. On the insurance side, the medical director or chief medical officer is involved heavily in all decisions made. In the pharmaceutical industry, physicians guide everything from strategy to clinical trials. Physicians all have a common view of the world that comes from four years of medical school learning how the human body works and what happens when that fabulous machine goes awry. Their view is also often informed by several years of postgraduate clinical training. This often decade-long experience changes the way these individuals think about the world and particularly about healthcare.

The extensive training is not just about learning the rigors of the profession. It is also designed to make physicians feel confident about decision making. We think that we are expert in matters far beyond our clinical training—and this sometimes leads to great challenges. Physicians are also taught to be conservative and cautious. We take the Hippocratic Oath ("First do no harm") quite seriously. Our training teaches us that workflows and routines are sacred. Mastering repetitive tasks enables us to work long hours and minimize the chance of error. These traits (confidence, conservatism and respect for routine) make most physicians very resistant to innovations that touch the care process.

The mystique around the knowledge—all nonphysicians view the knowledge base as scared and mystical—creates an environment in the healthcare industry where we are constantly needing approval from these confident, conservative, risk-averse, change-resistant and in-charge professionals.

And we wonder why healthcare changes so slowly.

"CHANGE CAN BE BRUTAL"

As someone who has been a promoter of disruptive technologies, I have often found myself in the position of having to sell new ideas to my colleagues. It is no easy task. About 15 years ago, I demoed a software application we had developed to a group of dermatologists. It would allow a nondermatologist, such as a primary care doctor or other frontline provider, to upload images of a patient's skin along with some of that person's medical history. Using this technology, an offsite dermatologist could enter a diagnosis and treatment recommendation on the same website. I was excited about this breakthrough because it was a smart and efficient way to cut costs and maintain quality. But I was greeted with a great deal of skepticism among some of the dermatologists in the group, including one who accused me of "cheapening our specialty."

At the time, I was reminded of this insightful observation from *The Prince* by Machiavelli: "It must be considered that there is nothing more difficult to carry out, nor more doubtful of success, nor more dangerous to handle, than to initiate a new order of things. For the reformer has enemies in all those who profit by the old order, and only lukewarm defenders in all those who would profit by the new order . . ."

Over the years, the tide has turned. Dermatologists (as well as other specialists) now share digital images and other clinical information via email and various social networks thousands of times a day. In fact, the American Academy of Dermatology has officially sponsored a teledermatology software application that members can use to provide volunteer services to underserved clinics. Hence, what once seemed threatening and intrusive to many dermatologists has now become an accepted part of the practice of medicine.

The reality is, change can be very unsettling, or as Partners' Dr. Gregg Meyer says bluntly, "Change can be brutal. If you ask me what my primary role is at Partners HealthCare, my official title is chief clinical officer, but what do I do every day? It's change management. That's my job. It's to get people to understand why we need to change, what's in it for them."

Meyer notes that it's very difficult for physicians and nurses to change how they have been trained to deal with patients. But, he also says, "The reality for most of my colleagues is that, with rare exception, if you say that this is a better way to take care of patients, they will come around to it."

Similarly, Steve R. Ommen, MD, associate dean at the Center for Connected Care at the Mayo Clinic in Rochester, Minnesota, remarks, "Providers will come to see that incorporating connected care into clinical practice will be of benefit to both their practice and their patients, *but it's not the way we've all been trained to practice medicine for 150 years.*"

For anyone looking for the comfort of the status quo, medicine today is a poor career choice. There has been a tremendous amount of tumult in the profession over the past decade and there's probably a lot more to come before the dust settles and a better, more efficient patient-centric system is in place. Unfortunately, medical school education is not keeping pace with these changes and many physicians are shell-shocked by the reality of today's demands on healthcare providers.

This epidemic of what I like to call "the new white coat anxiety" is reflected in the fact that many physicians have serious misgivings about how medicine is practiced today. According to the 2012 Physicians Foundation Survey, 84% feel that the medical profession is "in decline." A full 60% would retire today if they could afford to and, even more alarmingly, would switch to concierge medicine or reduce patient access to their services within the next one to three years. More to the point, close to 92% of physicians are unsure "where the health system will be or how they will fit into it three to five years from now," says the same survey.

If this proves to be true—if the majority of doctors are either leaving healthcare or refusing to accept insurance—it will put an even greater strain on a system that is trying to cope with millions of the newly insured and tens of millions of aging adults. It is the strongest argument yet for transforming a system that relies heavily on in-person, face-to-face care.

Susan Lane of Partners blames the incredibly packed schedules of most providers as a major source of the new white coat anxiety. Her credentials, RN, MSN, MBA, mean that Lane has been on both sides of the fence—practice and administration. She is also a practicing wellness clinician with a deep knowledge of complementary medicine.

Lane's own experiences working as a nurse have given her a unique insight into the stressful day-to-day lives of frontline practitioners. "A primary care doctor is expected to see a new patient every 15 minutes. During that time, she's supposed to take a history, write down notes, diagnose and in some cases prescribe a course of treatment," Lane says. "In between patient exams, the physician is being interrupted by phone calls and the unscheduled emergency that inevitably crops up during the day. So she's frantic about how to fit everything in."

And then, as Lane explains it, her administrator—who's being pressured by her bosses to improve efficiency—may come by and tell the physician that she should try to shave another minute off each visit so she can see an extra patient every hour.

"This is what physicians hate about practicing medicine," Lane emphasizes.

THE SOURCE OF ANGST

How did the physician's lot get this bad? Dr. Sandeep Jauhar, who is quoted at the start of this chapter, writes eloquently in his *Wall Street Journal* article about the "golden age" of American medicine in the mid-twentieth century when "doctors set their own hours and determined their own fees." It was a time when television shows like *Marcus Welby* and *General Hospital* depicted doctors who were "overwhelmingly positive, almost heroic."

In that essay, which was based on his 2014 book, *Doctored: The Disillusionment of an American Physician*, Jauhar cites a litany of complaints that he hears from his fellow physicians. Not surprisingly, doctors feel that they're drowning in paperwork and resent the amount of time they have to spend filling out insurance forms. They don't like feeling pressured to order extra tests or medical procedures to help boost a hospital administrator's bottom line. They are also sick and tired, writes Jauhar, of "the fear of lawsuits; runaway malpractice-liability premiums; and finally the loss of professional autonomy that has led many physicians to view themselves as pawns in a battle between insurers and the government."

His solution, however, is not to roll back the clock to the "good old days" before managed care and cost containment, but to quickly move forward with new business models. Says Jauhar, "We need systems that don't simply reward high-volume care but also help restore the humanism in doctor-patient relationships that has been weakened by business considerations, corporate directives and third-party intrusions."

This is a really important point, and as far as I'm concerned, one of the best arguments for connected health. Connected health enables new payment models by giving providers the tools, like remote patient monitoring and data analytics, to better manage their high-risk populations.

Liberated from fee-for-service, physicians can rethink how to deliver the best, most efficient care to a population. The tools include, but are not limited to, face-to-face visits. Connected health will enable physicians to work face-to-face with the few patients who really need that kind of attention and better manage patients with chronic conditions who often don't need repeat office visits. The one caveat, as I remind my team at Partners Connected Health, is in addition to maintaining high quality of care, the patients must feel cared for. In turn, doctors must not feel overwhelmed by the increased patient panel size.

BAIT AND SWITCH

Just like our healthcare system is mismatched with the problems confronting it today, I would argue that today's medical school education provides inadequate training for practice in the real world. Although there is talk of changing the curriculum, for the most part physicians are not taught to work in teams, as they inevitably will have to in the context of population health management. There is almost no training on remote patient monitoring and other health technologies, which will be a major part of practice within the next few years. And medical school education is still based on episodic, in-person interactions with patients, which have proven to be ineffective in managing the growing epidemic of chronic diseases. When new physicians embark on their careers, they find a broken healthcare system struggling to meet the needs of patients who require a great deal more attention than they can give in a brief office encounter.

As Dr. John Moore of Twine Health, whom I quoted at the beginning of the last chapter, observes, "The system was built around the idea of patients just coming in when they were sick. What we're dealing with now are the kinds of diseases where people need much more help, more often and much more efficiently." The company's product, Twine, is a cloud-based chronic care platform built on a shared healthcare record that facilitates a real-time, meaningful collaboration between patients, providers and care coordinators.

During a residency in ophthalmology, Moore was disillusioned by the fact that he was spending more time "face-to-face" with his patients inputting data into a computer than actually talking with them. In 2009, he joined Media Lab's New Media Medicine Group at MIT to focus on designing better healthcare technology that would facilitate more and better interaction between patients and physicians, as well as ways to monitor patients outside of the office.

"Patients have their own tracking devices and apps, but it's not in any way connected to their doctors or other clinicians," Moore says. "Clinicians have electronic medical records, but they're not in any way connected to their patients. So, they're both left pounding away at keyboards, or inputting data, but there's no collaboration happening between patient and provider."

This gets to another sore point among many physicians—electronic medical records. As far as I'm concerned, you can't have a truly integrated healthcare system in which you freely share data without them. This is not to say that EMRs can't be a lot better than they currently are (I am a curious mix of dreamer and pragmatist and when I talk about EMRs I'm more on the pragmatist side). They are poorly designed and lack interoperability, and they add time to most physicians' days. We need to work on these shortcomings, but the good that EMRs have done far outweighs the remaining challenges.

I can remember the days when patients would show up at my clinic and we could find no record in the hospital medical records room. There were instances where the record showed up but the physician notes were indecipherable and/or the lab pages tattered and/or crucial information missing. I also remember when we first made the migration from paper to electronic, I was pretty aggravated by the fact that I had to add a full two hours of time to each of my clinic sessions.

But I also recall the day that I was in my car driving home when my head nurse called about a patient. We talked about a certain medication regimen for this person's skin problem and as we were talking she was putting the prescription in the system. She then said, "There is an alert popping up reminding us to dose this drug differently because the patient has kidney failure." We changed the dose, she sent the prescription electronically to the pharmacy and the patient's condition improved. This story captures the value of our current generation of EMRs: They have facilitated in-the-moment decision making, electronic prescribing, provider decision support (the warning) and improved quality of care. In fact, without that warning my nurse and I could have had a significant medical error on our hands.

DATA ANXIETY

Although rapid advances in technology have made remote consultations and diagnosis both feasible and practical, there is still a great deal of apprehension and misunderstanding about the concept of virtual care. First, there is concern over the sheer amount of data we can collect and what to do with it. Mayo Clinic's Steve Ommen notes, "The amount of data we're going to be able to collect on an individual's physiology will be incredible, but we don't yet have the tools to make it meaningful for people. I think it will happen eventually, but it's going to be difficult."

Ommen also notes that more and more patients are coming into their doctors' appointments with their own devices and apps, like activity trackers, wireless blood pressure cuffs and glucometers. These devices store data in the cloud and enable users to share their information with whomever they like via email or social media. But people are often disappointed when physicians don't want to even see their self-collected data because, in reality, physicians have no way of making sense of this information in its current form.

"If you have a wireless blood pressure monitor, a physician needs to understand the device you're using and how to respond if we get an abnormal value," Ommen explains. "If it comes back 200/100, a physician doesn't want to send you a text telling you to call 911; they need to be able to say to the patient, 'Let's sit down and take it again.' Then, if it meets certain parameters, maybe you're fine, or maybe a nurse contacts you at some point. We still haven't figured out how to deal with this data. We have to understand the precision and the fail rate of the data so that we can respond in a way that's truly helpful."

Providers are even wary about data collected through hospital-based programs. Instead of viewing connected health as a way of liberating them from unnecessary interactions, many clinicians fear that it will be even more intrusive. They envision themselves tethered to a monitor, eyes glued to their screens, spending their days (and nights) reviewing a constant stream of patient data. They worry that they will be liable for tracking the lives of their patients 24/7, that their malpractice insurance will skyrocket, and that patients will be calling their office in the middle of the night because they see a fluctuation in their readings that is perfectly normal.

"We hear this concern from our practitioners at Partners all the time, but it's simply not true," says Susan Lane. "We explain that they are not responsible for watching their patients' data constantly and we make patients aware of this when they sign the consent form to be part of a connected health program."

The reality is, we have very clear consent language for patients, reminding them that connected health is not a substitute for 911. We use frontline, nonphysician providers to do the monitoring. These are folks that, as part of the new team-based, patient-centered medical home model of care that I mentioned earlier, have responsibility for a particular population of patients that they track closely using our systems. Doctors have access to the data if a decision needs to be made about medication management or if they wish to utilize it at the time of a visit. In the future, we'll be able to use decision support software to take large data sets (like thousands of blood pressure readings) and create insights that enable better care and also free providers from having to look at an excessive number of normal readings.

Partners has been a pioneer in remote patient monitoring, which is offered in a number of primary care practices throughout our network. The remotely monitored data—including blood pressure, blood glucose and weight—is easily viewable within the Partners' medical record system, giving our clinicians a more complete picture of a patient's condition. But no one is looking at the collected data every second of every day. A nurse, pharmacist or other provider will often first review the data and, if there is a problem, intervene appropriately and, if necessary, contact the physician.

Once a remote monitoring program is integrated into clinical practice, providers' initial concerns typically fade away and they begin to quickly see the benefits. "Practitioners see that it's not disruptive to what they're doing. In fact, most tell us that the data gives them better insight into their patients, and they feel that they are providing better care. Providers actually feel good about this new delivery model and want to work this way with more patients," Lane notes.

DEBUNKING SOME MYTHS

Despite the fact that healthcare is moving toward a connected health model, many physicians cling to the belief that in-person interaction with patients is always superior and that their own observational skills are equal to—if not better than—technology. Among many providers there is an almost visceral fear of automation, a deep-seated belief that hands-on care is always the best. They have an absolute conviction that the move to a more efficient healthcare system runs counter to the practice of "the art of medicine."

Physicians and nurses are trained to believe that they must do their own evaluation, take their own patient history, perform their own exams and even do their own imaging/lab studies. This mindset leads to redundancy of testing, more visits and follow-up visits and even more testing, which not only eats up time, but accounts for huge waste. This also makes it hard to realize the vision of a single electronic health record where data is shared among providers. It is one of the primary reasons why waiting rooms are overflowing with patients, doctors feel so rushed and patients feel that they're being short-changed. What's even worse, there's no evidence that anybody is getting any healthier because of it.

I would argue that, in many cases, much of what we automatically assume must be done face-to-face can be done just as well through automation and connected health. In other words, physicians or nurses don't necessarily have to be in the same room with patients to gather data, make a diagnosis or even dole out advice.

I'm not suggesting that we will ever do away with face-to-face interaction. There's no dispute that an acute situation that requires hands-on treatment needs to be in person. A televisit or remote EKG on a smartphone isn't the way to treat a heart attack, stitch up a deep cut or set a broken limb. There are also times when face-to-face encounters may be important if just to deal with the emotional gravity of a situation. But for the most part, the management of most chronic diseases can be done very well—if not better—using connected health technologies. I know that this is a provocative statement bound to elicit disbelief from some of my peers, but hear me out.

Think of interactions with a healthcare provider as falling into two categories: (1) diagnostic/assessment and (2) education/caring. The foundation of diagnosis and assessment is the medical history and physical exam: This is part of data gathering. Some providers feel that their gestalt or intuition when seeing the patient in person and doing a hands-on physical exam is infinitely more important than any lab tests or imaging results. This may have been true 50 years ago, but it's no longer the case. Although we now have the tools to gather vital signs remotely, many doctors will argue that they are not as accurate as those collected in person. Today better sensors and data science are making that argument obsolete.

For the most part, I challenge the basic assumption that most components of a diagnosis and assessment need to be done in person. In fact, it may make more sense not to.

For example, is it really necessary to take a patient history at the time of an office visit? Oftentimes when a patient arrives for an appointment, she is handed a clipboard with a form to fill out. Then, the doctor and patient review her answers. But in this day and age, it makes much more sense for the patient's history to be taken online, which she can even do at home. An electronic questionnaire has one major advantage over a paper form: The online questionnaire can use branching logic that refines questions based on previous answers. The information can then be automatically sent to the patient's medical record so that all of her doctors have access to it. I think it's pretty clear that allowing the patient to fill out the questionnaire at her own pace, at home or at work, is better than collecting this information during the office visit. In most cases, if there are any gaps or questions, they can easily be resolved through email or texting—before the patient even arrives at the doctor's office. I'd say no contest here, automated is better than in-person.

The other part of data gathering is the actual physical exam. Some of you may be thinking, well of course, here is an area where the personal touch trumps technology. My response is, maybe not. We'd be hard pressed to say that the old way of listening to the lungs and heart with a stethoscope is more accurate than an echocardiogram or chest CT, or that palpating the abdomen is more accurate than an imaging study. My point is, we've moved beyond the point that human beings can do better than smart medical technology. At its best, the physical exam is a crude screening tool.

Of course, we're not going to order medical tests for everybody, but I think it's time that physicians lay to rest the "face-to-face is always better medicine" myth. It's just that—a self-perpetuating myth that reinforces our own importance.

Perhaps the biggest argument against the notion that "in person is better" is the fact that, despite all the hype about face-to-face care, a physician, on average, spends very little time with a patient. Even the patients who are "frequent flyers" get, in aggregate, one to two hours of face time with their doctor annually. Consider the fact that there are 8,760 hours in a year. Are we really saying we don't value measuring what goes on the 99% of time the patient is not in front of us? Of course not! Having a more complete picture of a patient's health using remote monitoring or self-generated data is an important component in improving the quality of our care and clinical outcomes.

Now, let's look at the education/caring part of patient management, which is admittedly trickier. Providers, and to a lesser extent patients, intuitively believe that quality care means meeting the doctor face-to-face. The main reason for this belief is that a trusting, caring relationship with a provider is thought to be a cornerstone of effective care. It is undoubtedly true that trust is critical for an effective relationship and that effective relationships with providers lead to improved care (the likely best explanation for the placebo effect). But, I want to call into question the assertion that a trusting relationship has to be human-to-human or face-to-face.

Many providers (particularly nurses) feel that they can better assess a patient's reaction to a diagnosis, as well as that person's understanding of what are often complicated concepts, along with the person's emotional involvement in the interaction, if meeting face-to-face. This is also the reason so many providers make their first leap into virtual care via video visits—they get the audio and video component of the interaction as opposed to just text.

It's not wrong to value face-to-face interactions with patients for all of the reasons noted here. But the more open-minded may wonder, "How much of the emotional value of the interaction is on the part of the provider rather than the patient?"

Providers are surrounded by stimuli that trick them into thinking everyone (staff, patients and colleagues) loves them. On the one hand, they are the revenue rainmakers of the operation and colleagues and staff respect that. On the other hand, they write prescriptions and order tests, so patients feel the need to always be nice too. This can lead to an "emperor wearing no clothes" phenomenon and a situation in which providers think that people are always eager to see them.

I LIKE "IT"

While it goes against the grain of what many physicians and nurses believe, our studies and the work of others show that most patients are just as comfortable working with a "relational agent," like an on-screen avatar, as they are with a real live person. In fact, many actually prefer it. I call this phenomenon "emotional automation." People may initially bristle at the concept of dealing with an avatar, and assume they'd prefer working with a flesh-and-blood human being, but that's because they're thinking about those annoying interactions with the automated interactive voice system when they call customer support or the poorly computerized voice in the parking garage where they pay their bill. These are unfortunate examples and we'll have to do much better in healthcare. The interesting thing, though, is that we don't have to be perfect. Many of us learn to trust and happily interact with relational agents every day.

We like to believe that individuals will simply not bond with a virtual presence as they would with a human being. Yet, there are numerous examples of how people get very attached to technology, oftentimes imparting human qualities to it. The entire premise of the wildly successful Tomagotchi Friends toys introduced in the 1990s was that children would love and nurture these handheld "digital pals" as they would a favorite family pet. As of 2010 (the latest figure I could find), there were some 79 million of these toys sold worldwide—clearly kids can become very attached to an electronic friend. And it's not just children forging relationships with "things." Adults have been known to grow so attached to automobile navigation systems that they assign them names! And millions of people consult Siri or Cortana even more frequently than they speak with their friends.

The late Clifford Nass wrote extensively about this phenomenon in his 2010 book, *The Man Who Lied to His Laptop*. Although we often joke about these relationships, to the people who are experiencing them, they feel very real.

Not surprisingly, the theme of human/relational agent love has already made it to the big screen. The 2013 romantic comedy *Her* by Spike Jonze explores the relationship between a human male, Theodore, and the computer operating system (OS) that he falls head over heels in love with. It may sound a bit wacky, but the OS system is portrayed by the very human voice of Scarlett Johansson and it is very believable. Unlike a real human girlfriend, the OS system, aka Samantha, is able to study Theodore's every move—and nearly every thought—through his online search history. This makes it possible for Samantha to anticipate what he needs precisely when he needs it, which no human being could do regardless of how intuitive she (or he) might be (or would even want to be). When the relationship fizzles at the end of the movie (Samantha gets bored with him), you can't help but feel that Theodore is experiencing a real sense of loss.

At Partners, we've explored different ways of using relational agents with our patients in different capacities. For example, we collaborated with Tim Bickmore, an associate professor at the College of Computer and Information Science at Northeastern University, to show that a Virtual Coach is powerful in terms of sustaining improved walking behavior in an experimental cohort. In this study, Karen, the Virtual Coach, simulated face-to-face conversation, including verbal and nonverbal communication, as well as goal setting, positive reinforcement, problem solving, education and social interaction. Dialogue was tailored based on the participant's progress, current status against their goals and interaction with the Virtual Coach, such as asking Karen a question or asking for help.

The study results showed a significant percentage increase in step count for participants with access to the Internet-based coaching developed by Bickmore, versus those without access to Karen. Just under 60% of participants working with Karen agreed that the avatar motivated them to be more active and almost 90% reported feeling guilty if they skipped an appointment with her. More to the point, those who had the three weekly meetings with Karen had significantly better daily step counts than control participants who only had access to their own activity tracker data.

Bickmore, who is a leader in the field of human interaction with relational agents, has done some intriguing work of his own. In one groundbreaking study, he showed that patients who are preparing to be discharged from a hospital actually *prefer* to get their discharge instructions from a computerized agent as opposed to a person. When asked why they favored the avatar over a human, patients typically responded, *"It doesn't talk down to me. It isn't in a hurry. I can think carefully about my questions and ask them as many times as I want without feeling judged."*

Of course, most doctors don't want to believe that patients may regard them as judgmental, or that some people may at times prefer working with an

"It" over an MD. This, along with all the other sweeping changes in healthcare that are driving it to become more efficient, may be very hard for some physicians to swallow. Their world is shifting beneath their feet and they feel very unsteady.

This discussion of "the new white coat anxiety" reminds me of a play by the absurdist British playwright Harold Pinter, who was among other things a playful linguist. In *The Birthday Party*, he confuses us many times with the meaning of the words up and down. A couple of lines I'll paraphrase involve one character referring to another who has not emerged from his upstairs bedroom in the morning. "Is he down, yet?" she asks. To which her counterpart replies, "I'm not sure if he's up." My point here is, many physicians working today are also not sure of what is down or up. Many went into a field thinking they'd help people, make a good living, be universally respected and be able to concentrate on their true value-adding training, "the medical stuff."

Today all of those things are in flux. Physicians are frustrated, harried and often annoyed, in addition to all of those traits I mentioned at the beginning of the chapter (confident, conservative and risk averse). Yet they are almost universally decision makers and we need them to move forward to this next exciting phase of healthcare delivery.

SELLING DISRUPTION

This chapter is merely a primer. But armed with the knowledge of the challenges that the early twenty-first-century physician faces, and understanding a bit more about sales psychology, should enable you to move your innovation forward faster.

So how do you make a sale to a doctor, particularly when the product or service is new and potentially disruptive?

- Communicate with utmost respect. Rightly or not, providers expect to be treated with deference. Everyone around them in healthcare already does, so you will have to as well.
- Don't try to pull the wool over their eyes. These are highly educated, highly skeptical individuals who pride themselves on their BS filter.

- Come with data. The pharmaceutical salesperson will tell you that he wins the doctor over in a few minutes with two time-honored tools, a reprint and a bar chart. Doctors will ask for the evidence base behind your innovation and will be very critical of that piece, so be ready.
- Forget the "tchotchkes." The old-fashioned persuasion tools of free food and other goodies are falling out of favor. Some MDs are forbidden from taking gifts and even those who are not are tentative because of the Sunshine Act and their fear of online reporting of their gifts.
- Be persistent. The sales cycle is long and MDs pride themselves on making you work for the sale—it will probably take many meetings.
- Do your best to make any new product or service advantageous to them. Will it improve patient care? Will it enable them to look better in front of their patients? Will it enable them to make or save money? Will it lighten their workload?
- Keep your pitch brief and to the point. Time is of the essence.

6

Some Healthy Disruption

"Starting with baby boomers, there's an attitudinal shift where convenience is often more valued than traditional relationships. The new way of thinking is, 'It doesn't matter whether it's my healthcare or my banking services, I want it now and I want it to be convenient!'"

—Harry L. Leider, MD, MBA, chief medical officer and group vice president, Walgreens

"Younger vets expect to do everything online like they do with other goods and services—update addresses, reorder a prescription, make an appointment, get information and change their mailing preferences. We have to get all of that right: It is part of the foundation of connected health."

—Neil Evans, MD, co-director of Connected Health, Office of Informatics and Analytics, Veterans Health Administration, and practicing primary care internist, Veterans Affairs Medical Center

In January 2015, I received a letter from my primary care physician alerting me that I needed to get blood drawn prior to my upcoming appointment.

Without that information, he had no way of knowing whether the statin drug I was taking was managing my cholesterol effectively. Hence, it made perfect sense to complete the lab work ahead of time so that my doctor could discuss any changes in my treatment plan during our appointment. The only problem was the notice for the lab work arrived in my mailbox on January 17—*two days after my appointment on January 15*.

Considering the inconvenience and inefficiency of this system, sending reminders in the mail—in 2015—is just puzzling. Today, 90% of Americans have mobile phones, more than 80% send or receive text messages and more than half receive and send email. I'm sure many of you are thinking, "Well, this kind of thing happens all the time, what do you expect?" That's my point. It does happen all the time and it's indicative of a healthcare infrastructure that has had great difficulty keeping up with the times. In this day and age, I—and I believe most other people—have come to expect a lot more. For all the talk of the "consumerization" of healthcare, there has been very little of it happening within conventional healthcare systems.

Perhaps the most forward thinking attempts to create a "consumer-centric" health experience are coming from organizations not encumbered by archaic payment models or paralyzed by the "we've always done it this way" bias. Later in this chapter, I will describe how two very different organizations—the Veterans Health Administration (VHA), the biggest healthcare provider in the United States, and Walgreens, America's largest pharmacy chain, which also operates some 400-plus walk-in clinics—are using technology to provide a better consumer experience and ultimately better care. Both the VHA and Walgreens have responded to the new healthcare marketplace with bold ideas; in their own unique way, each is beginning to create a new model of what a "seamless" healthcare system could look like.

From my perspective, I see a reluctance—or inertia—on the part of most providers to make necessary changes to improve the healthcare experience for consumers. As discussed in Chapter 5, there may be many reasons for this, but at the top of my list is the unique position doctors have in both the decision making around care delivery and the capture of revenue in the business model. This creates a culture that is slower to change than any I know of. It sets up scenarios where a hospital, clinic or practice may offer state-of-the-art, highly sophisticated diagnostic tests and high-tech operating rooms, but its interaction with consumers and patients is oftentimes stuck in midcentury America.

I have a distinct memory of a trip to the family physician when I was growing up in the early sixties. I had some kind of stomach bug. My parents and I sat in the waiting room of my doctor's first floor office. He brought me in, took a history, examined me, discussed his findings with my parents and wrote out a prescription. On our way to the pharmacy, we stopped at the bank and my dad waited in line to cash his paycheck. We also stopped to get our gas tank filled by a uniformed man who offered to wash the windshield and check the oil. The last stop before the pharmacy was to pick up maps and an itinerary for our summer driving trip from a local travel agent.

In 2015, only one of those experiences has changed very little—and you probably know which one. The bank, the gas station and the travel agency have all been disrupted by technology. We withdraw cash from an ATM and I can deposit my paycheck by snapping a picture of it with my iPhone. We pump our own gas and book our trips on Expedia, Travelocity and other travel sites, download a boarding pass and check into the airport by swiping the screen on a smartphone. The only thing that has remained pretty much the same is the patient experience of having to visit a physician's office or clinic for care.

IF YOU DON'T KNOW ME BY NOW

There's also an annoying—at times unsettling—unpredictability to the consumer healthcare experience. A patient never knows what to expect. Sometimes the doctor's office will call, email or text ahead to remind you of an appointment, sometimes it doesn't. Sometimes you can access your lab results online; sometimes not. And, almost never can you do meaningful work online with your provider; in most cases, anything important is still done face-to-face. The medical office may be top-heavy with personnel to manage patient visits, yet most patient conditions are chronic and require day-to-day lifestyle monitoring and intervention.

But having all these receptionists, lab technicians, nurses and other staff is not making the experience any better for patients and consumers. The check-in process at most clinics and hospitals is cumbersome and decades outmoded. Patients are repeatedly asked to fill out the same forms that they filled out before, even though the information is often already in their medical records. Perhaps I've become spoiled by my interactions with companies that understand how to create a positive and frictionless experience for consumers, actually making the interaction enjoyable. These companies make you feel as if they "know" you and care about your preferences. You know what to expect when you navigate their websites and you get the sense that they've been waiting for you to return—with open arms. Amazon knows my taste in books; Zappos knows my preference in shoes; Soap.com knows my past purchases and periodically reminds me when it's time to reorder from my previous list; Netflix keeps track of the programs that I've watched.

My healthcare provider is certainly keeping track of what medications I'm taking, what tests I've had and my medical problems, but this is not information easily available to me. And why can't my provider alert me via text or email when I have an upcoming appointment, tell me how to prepare for the appointment and provide important information like where to get my lab work done? I guess my question is, if it's a simple matter of reviewing my blood test results, why do I even need to do this in person, face-to-face? Why do I have to take time off from work to see my doctor? Wouldn't a virtual visit or even an email exchange suffice for routine things?

For much of its modern history, healthcare has taken the "seller's market" approach. The thinking is, "You need us more than we need you." It worked for an older generation that had a reverence for doctors and for insurance companies that covered most, if not all, of their healthcare bills. That generation is being replaced by the new healthcare consumer, the one who "wants it now" and who, by the way, is probably paying a high deductible and copay, and expects to get more for his or her money.

Walgreens is ready and willing to provide that "on-demand" service in a brick-and-mortar and digital setting, a sign that this iconic retailer sees a future that extends well beyond its current tagline, "At the corner of happy & healthy," into the world of connected health. In fact, companies like Walgreens, CVS and Walmart are poised to play an even greater role in healthcare, largely by offering an improved customer experience.

I will tell the story of Walgreens in depth here, but the others are similar in some respects. The most important point of the Walgreens example is how today's consumers can envision a world that allows them to exercise choice and benefit from enhanced convenience in the way they access various healthcare services. This is a crack in the armor of the doctor monopoly.

CHANGING THE PARADIGM

Over the past few years, Walgreens has introduced a number of forward-thinking initiatives that have positioned it as much more than a community pharmacy. It is now a model for a consumer-friendly and consumer-centric healthcare provider and partner for the digital age. Its industry-leading programs include an affordable telemedicine option for virtual doctor consultations, a loyalty program that provides incentives for consumers to track activities online or through personal health devices, and 400-plus walk-in Healthcare Clinics nationwide. With consumer convenience in mind, Walgreens also recently partnered with Theranos, the revolutionary Silicon Valley startup that created a technology that enables comprehensive blood testing from a small drop of blood cheaper and faster than conventional labs.

With these and other innovations under development, Walgreens is poised to benefit from four converging trends: the shortage of primary care physicians; the need for providers in higher-risk payment models to promote wellness and produce better outcomes; a rapidly growing number of seniors with increased healthcare needs; and a younger, newly insured population that places a high value on convenience and mobility.

What began as a corner pharmacy in 1901—and is credited with inventing the malted milk shake—is now part of Walgreens Boots Alliance, Inc. (WBA), a Deerfield, Illinois–based global enterprise that owns Walgreens, Duane Reade drug stores (primarily located in the New York City metropolitan area), Boots (a European retail pharmacy), and other pharmacy-related healthcare businesses. Walgreens alone operates more than 8,200 pharmacies in the United States.

About a decade ago, faced with growing competition from online retailers like Amazon, more cost-conscious consumers and reimbursement pressures that were beginning to impact profit margins within the industry, Walgreens was at a crossroads. According to Alexandra Jung, former senior vice president of Walgreens Health Services (a division of the company that has since been sold), in an interview published in *Progressions 2012* on ey.com, "The nation's largest drug store chain decided to extend its business model deeply into the provider space, fundamentally reinventing itself by focusing on establishing partnerships to improve health care delivery and patient outcomes." (Jung is now a partner and principal with Ernst & Young.)

A first step was the 2007 acquisition of Take Care Health Systems, a retail clinic provider. What began as a 50-clinic operation now encompasses more than 400 Walgreens Healthcare Clinics chainwide, typically staffed by licensed family nurse practitioners. The clinics offer consumers a wide range of nonemergency services, including immunizations, wellness visits, camp and school physicals, health screenings, testing for conditions like diabetes and high blood pressure, and treatments for assorted aches, pains, sprains and minor injuries. These walk-in clinics tend to attract a younger clientele and about 40% of clinic users don't have their own primary care physician. Although most insurance plans are accepted, the cost of seeing a nurse practitioner is significantly less than the typical $100 or so fee for a doctor visit, making Walgreens Healthcare Clinics an appealing option for many individuals who have to pay high deductibles and copays.

Another real benefit is that a patient's records (including prescriptions) can be accessed from any Healthcare Clinic in the Walgreens system, which eliminates the constant and annoying process of filling out forms. Consumers also have the option of making appointments online or dropping in.

When Walgreens and other retailers (like CVS MinuteClinic) opened their doors in the early 2000s, there was some talk in the medical community that these cheaper and more convenient purveyors of health would steal patients from doctors, cutting into the bottom line. In a truly defensive mode, now 15 years later, many healthcare systems are operating their own version of these clinics, often focused on urgent care. The outcome of this battle for acute care is still unclear. Both CVS and Walgreens have forged some significant partnerships with hospitals, health systems and community health organizations throughout the United States including, for Walgreens, Northwestern Memorial Hospital in Chicago, and physician groups affiliated with the Johns Hopkins Health System.

To be sure, Walgreens Healthcare Clinics offer convenience, but that certainly isn't the secret sauce that potentially gives the company an edge. Its main competitor, CVS, actually has twice as many MinuteClinics in its stores throughout the country, and has plans to expand. Further, urgent care centers that provide even more extensive care (like onsite x-rays) are popping up on just about every street corner and in every mall in America. What these in-pharmacy care centers offer is a jumping off point for any number of other services.

REWARDING HEALTHY BEHAVIOR

What makes Walgreens a trailblazer in healthcare is not what the chain is doing with its brick-and-mortar stores, but the creative ways that it's using digital health to drive consumer loyalty, extend its reach and fill an important treatment gap in the healthcare system.

Although Walgreens was one of the last big chain retailers to start a consumer loyalty program, launching its Balance Rewards Program in 2012, it has moved beyond the standard points-for-purchase model. The company's unique *Balance Rewards for healthy choices*® program enables consumers to earn rewards points for participating in fitness and wellness programs and activities, and accrue points for setting and meeting health and wellness goals. Consumers have a choice of inputting data manually or—and this is where it gets really interesting—syncing compatible wearable trackers, health devices and fitness apps to their Balance Rewards account. The program also rewards behaviors like refilling a prescription, which can be done by scanning the prescription barcode using the Walgreens mobile app. And Walgreens continues to anticipate the needs of its customers. Recently, the pharmacy launched its

Walgreens app designed exclusively for Apple Watch and will also be integrating its Balance Rewards program with Apple Pay.

For those who want more support, Walgreens offers Your Digital Health Advisor powered by WebMD, an automated digital coaching platform with cobranded digital health and wellness content that is not available on the regular WebMD site. For example, this program enables consumers to set goals to lose weight, exercise more, quit smoking or control asthma or diabetes. People who use the integrated WebMD tools can also earn Balance Rewards points for inputting their data and making progress.

Right now, about 400,000 people each month are syncing their devices and apps to earn Balance Rewards points. Granted, it's just a start considering that Walgreens had an astonishing 86 million Balance Rewards members as of May 2015. But as the popularity of tracking grows, it makes sense that consumer use of this program will also grow.

Offering points for better health and increased activity is not just a great way to build brand loyalty; it will also provide some fascinating data that could be useful in many different ways. For example, as you learn about people's health behaviors, you can link this information to their product preferences and prescription needs. This data also provides greater insight into the impact of lifestyle on product choices and health status, and will create opportunities to provide consumers with tailored healthcare solutions, services and products. And, as a side benefit, consumers who earn points this way probably feel that Walgreens really cares about them and their progress. It builds a stronger bond.

Recently, Walgreens moved into a new arena—virtual chronic care management support. Using Qualcomm Life's 2net Platform, Balance Rewards members are able to sync compatible blood pressure cuffs, glucose monitors and weight scales to their rewards account, and give pharmacists electronic access to their biometric data and health status information. A few years ago, something like this might have been dismissed as a good idea that lacked a business model. Today, in the era of population health management, value-based payments and penalties for hospital readmissions, this model has a good chance for success.

Dr. Harry Leider, chief medical officer of Walgreens, whom I quoted at the start of this chapter, predicts that "Forward thinking health systems will invest in these services to support patients with common chronic illnesses, and Walgreens can be a big part of the solution." And he adds, "Since a huge part of managing chronic illness is medication adherence, we also think our pharmacists can play a major role here."

Leider also notes that chronically ill people spend a great deal of time in Walgreens stores interacting with pharmacists and other healthcare staff. For example, the typical diabetes patient visits a Walgreens pharmacy, on average, *20 times* a year. That, combined with consumer-generated data, gives Walgreens a great deal more knowledge of a patient's everyday lifestyle and habits than a doctor who typically sees the patient two or three times a year.

"Walgreens stores have two big levers," says Leider. "One, we know when patients don't pick up their medication—we have that data. The doctors in hospitals or medical practices often don't have this information on a real-time basis. We know it because we create automatic alerts when our customers don't fill their prescription on time. Number two, because these chronically ill patients are in our community pharmacies frequently, we have a significant and trusted relationship with them."

Leider also points out that if patients aren't taking their medications, pharmacists are in a position to intervene immediately. "If they're not adhering to the medication regimen, our pharmacists can work with the patients to figure out why," he says. "Is it confusion because they have to take so many pills? Is it side effects? Is it financial? Is it a belief that they don't think the medication is doing any good? Is it making them dizzy when they stand up? We can find out why and try to help."

In 2010, Walgreens launched Pharmacy Chat, a 24/7 service that allows users to interact in a live online chat with members of its pharmacy staff. A partnership with MDLIVE in 2014 also enables Walgreens consumers to book a virtual appointment or meet immediately via a video conference with a board certified physician, through a website, or using an app, for $49 per visit. Walgreens offers this service in 13 states, with plans to expand to 25 states by the end of 2015. Given the low price tag of this telemedicine visit, Leider admits that this service isn't a big money maker. Rather, it's more about building loyalty and, in the process, more traffic to the pharmacy. "The people who are accessing this through Walgreens are going to be more connected to us from a brand loyalty perspective as it builds on our historic value proposition of providing convenient and trusted care and products," he explains. "Patients can utilize any pharmacy, but a significant number of the prescriptions generated by telemedicine are likely to come to Walgreens to get filled."

IF YOU LIKE US, YOU'LL GIVE US YOUR DATA

On top of it all, Walgreens is still investing in brick-and-mortar pharmacies and newer flagship stores in places like Boston, San Francisco, Washington, DC, and Los Angeles. The goal is to attract Gen Xers and millennials—younger, hipper consumers who value both convenience and a shopping experience that is more personalized than ordering online.

Shelf upon shelf packed with the necessities of life, an extensive fresh food market (including, if you come at the right time, an onsite sushi chef) and a walk-in medical clinic are the winning formula for the Walgreens-owned Duane Reade located at 40 Wall Street in Lower Manhattan. This fancier, upscale version of the typical pharmacy/retailer gets four stars on Yelp, which is a real accomplishment considering how picky New Yorkers can be.

The store is a huge expanse, brightly lit, uncluttered and very appealing. You enter the space via an escalator from the marble lobby. The first thing you see is a rack of healthy snacks, including packages of nuts and energy bars; a few feet away is a well-stocked fresh foods department. As you move deeper into the space, you pass aisles stocked with just about every consumer item you could possibly need, from hair dryers, hosiery and reading glasses to the latest magazines and bathroom scales.

Eventually, you get to Duane Reade's walk-in clinic, DR Walk-In Medical Care, a compact area with two private rooms (so you don't have to have your shots or blood pressure taken in public) and a waiting area outside. As the informational brochure explains, prescriptions are written when it is "clinically appropriate" and consumers can fill them at any pharmacy they choose. The DR Walk-In clinic, however, is strategically located just a few feet away from the Duane Reade pharmacy, which has a comfortable waiting area with chairs and a few desktop computers for customer use. Close by are displays for products for diabetes care, first aid and foot care. I would guess very few people actually take those prescriptions to another pharmacy—why would they? And I would also wager that while people are waiting to have their prescriptions filled, they suddenly remember that they need to stock up on a few items for their medicine cabinet or refrigerator. It starts to look hopeless for traditional hospital systems to compete with this! An experience as pleasant and convenient as this will make you want to return and likely incentivize consumers to apply for a rewards card. And pretty soon, some of those younger shoppers will be syncing their activity trackers and apps—and their data—to earn points for their healthy choices.

The Walgreens story gives us a blueprint for how businesses might disrupt traditional healthcare delivery and do so in a way that improves consumer experience. Watch the company carefully for ideas on how your own business can do this.

CONNECTING TO VETERANS

Another reason why traditional healthcare has been so slow to respond to changing times and why it hasn't become more consumer focused has to do with the economics that drive the business. With that in mind, let's take an in-depth look at a healthcare system that is not encumbered by arcane and bizarre economics: the Veterans Health Administration system.

The Veterans Health Administration (VHA), under the direction of the U.S. Department of Veterans Affairs (VA), runs the largest integrated health system in the United States, consisting of 150 medical centers, 1,400 community-based out-patient clinics, community living centers, Vet Centers and "domiciliaries" or in-home care facilities. Despite all of its real estate around the country, in the world of connected health, VHA has been a bold pioneer and innovator. In a statement issued last fall, Veterans Affairs secretary Robert A. McDonald said that telehealth is one of the areas they have identified for growth, explaining that "a brick-and-mortar facility is not the only option for healthcare."

VA is proving that to be true on a massive scale. In 2014, VHA treated 690,000 Veterans via telemedicine, allowing individuals to get treatment in their own homes or in facilities close to home while providing remote access to necessary specialists. VA also offers real-time video consultation that covers 44 clinical specialties including TelePrimary Care, TeleMental Health, TeleCardiology, TeleNeurology, Women's Telehealth, TeleAmputation Clinics, TeleAudiology, Home Telehealth care and case management of chronic conditions. VA Store-and-Forward Telehealth enables providers to receive and store clinical images so that a specialist can analyze them remotely, providing specialty care anywhere a patient may live.

Equally impressive is the fact that nearly 160,000 Veterans across the United States identified as high risk are using home monitors to gather data on various vital signs including pulse oximeter readings, blood pressure and diabetes glucose levels. This data is reviewed remotely by a care coordinator who can intervene if necessary.

Other providers have had to figure out ways to squeeze telehealth into rigid payment models—a classic square peg in a round hole problem. But as both the payer and provider for a sizable number of its patient population, VA has been freer to be more experimental. Out of the VHA's $56 billion budget for fiscal year 2016, $1.2 billion is earmarked for telehealth programs.

According to a report by Adam Darkins, MD, the VA's former chief consultant for Telehealth Services, the investment in telehealth is paying off. In 2013, VA telehealth services saved, on average, $1,999 per patient annually, and reduced bed days of care by 58% and hospital admissions by 35%. Remote clinical video telehealth services reduced hospitalizations among patients with mental health problems by 35%.

Good technology is the backbone of connected health—that's a given. But as we have learned at Partners Connected Health, even the best gadgets won't guarantee engagement. So it's not at all surprising to me that VHA's co-director of Connected Health, Neil C. Evans, whom I quoted at the start of this chapter, uses the word "relationship" frequently when he talks about the VA's telehealth program. "One of the things that we've learned over the past 15 to 20 years is that *relationships* really matter in healthcare," says Evans.

"Having a primary care provider who knows who you are, and who invests in you as a patient over the course of many years, is not just important from a patient standpoint, but from a quality standpoint. We think of connected health as a way to extend the trusted relationships that Veterans have with their VA health provider, beyond what that provider could deliver otherwise, simply by delivering care face-to-face."

Evans, who manages his own panel of 400 patients at the Veterans Affairs Medical Center in Washington, DC, notes that connected health was conceived to be an extension of the VA policy to proactively reach out to high-risk patients. "We asked ourselves, 'How do we take the idea of population health and create the tools whereby a patient can get what he needs to manage his condition right in his own home?'"

BRANCHING OUT

VA's interest in connected health extends beyond the potential cost savings. The reality is, the system is so vast and geographically expansive, it would be hard to exist without it. The Veterans Health Administration is responsible for delivering care across the entire United States, Alaska, Hawaii and all territories. In 2015, VA will offer care to an estimated 9.4 million enrollees, including 1.4 million Veterans from the Afghanistan and Iraq wars, aging Vietnam War baby boomers and elderly survivors of the Korean conflict and World War II. About 1.8 million of these enrollees will engage in some aspect of virtual care, either through telehealth, remote monitoring or use of VA's patient portal. About two out of five VA users are rural residents, of which 1.5% are described as "high rural," meaning they live in very isolated, often underserved areas.

Like the rest of the healthcare system, VHA is facing a number of challenges, including the epidemic of chronic disease and an aging population that requires more care. In addition, VA must provide care to address the special needs of Veterans returning home with both physical and psychological wounds from multiple tours of duty, a rapidly expanding population in certain communities.

All of this has put a strain on the system.

In recent years, Veterans Affairs has been the subject of scathing criticism, primarily due to long delays for scheduling appointments and follow-up care, especially in underserved medical communities and/or those that have attracted large numbers of aging retirees. Despite these problems, VHA, for the most part, gets very high grades among its users. Objective studies have shown that the quality of care VA offers is equal to, if not often better than, private health systems.

For example, when most providers were just talking about electronic health records, VA began work on developing its own, called VistA—Veterans Health Information Systems and Technology Architecture. By 2001, VA was 100% electronic. VA was also one of the first healthcare systems to use secure email to communicate with patients, a service that is usually not covered or poorly reimbursed by most payers.

"For us, this was a no brainer, as it enabled us to extend our reach," Evans explains. "Primary care teams across the system embraced 'desktop medicine,' where physicians, nurse practitioners and nurses deliver virtual care through telephone visits or secure messaging. This would be very difficult to do in a fee-for-service environment."

Today, more than 2.5 million Veterans use My HealtheVet, the next generation VistA personal health online record. This new system enables individuals to order prescription refills, view their electronic health record, including doctor's notes, imaging results and lab data, and through its special VA Blue Button feature, share information with non-VA providers and send secure messages to their VA healthcare team.

Though it is possible that the use of secure messaging might actually increase patients' visits and engagement with the VA healthcare system, Evans says it is a good thing. "I can tell you anecdotally that my patients who engage via connected health technologies are more informed and often easier to manage, because our interactions become much richer than simply one or two face-to-face meetings a year. We get little snippets of interactions over the course of a year, which allows for a more holistic interchange about their health. It also enhances the team-based approach to care. When a team nurse answers a secure email message, that nurse also becomes a trusted advisor to the patient." In fact, VA has published a study showing that implementation of secure messaging is associated with a reduction in utilization of Urgent Care.

To Evans, My Health*e*Vet is not just a way to automate interactions with the healthcare system, but also serves as an "entry into connected health," empowering patients to assume responsibility for the management of their own healthcare. "By getting people engaged, they understand that technology can be a very useful tool in health self-management," he says. "The simple act of clicking onto a website, reordering your prescription and two days later it's in your mailbox—that really changes your perception of what digital tools can do."

SOMETHING FOR EVERY GENERATION

As noted above, the VA population is incredibly diverse in just about every way, and includes World War II survivors (as of this writing, the oldest patient is 107) right up to the newest discharges from the Afghanistan and Iraq wars. Understandably, there is a huge gap among the different generations, in terms of their level of technological sophistication, as well as their expectations. Evans notes that younger Veterans want to be able to manage their health on their smartphones. "Increasingly, younger Veterans have the expectation that they will be able to transact with any organization they do business with online or on their mobile device, by whatever platform they choose to use," he says.

In contrast many older Veterans still want to be able to use technology in familiar ways, and VA offers them several different options. According to Evans, "Within our suite of technologies, we have wireless options for our more tech savvy patients. Some of our other patients value having a device in a fixed location that they can hook up to their landline—which they proudly maintain. They want to take their blood pressure sitting in their big chair in their home by their phone and we can do that for them," he says.

One shortcoming of the VA system is that Veterans can't book appointments online yet. Patients still have to call their healthcare facility to do that.

But there are pilot projects in the works testing mobile and web applications to allow Veterans to directly schedule their own appointments.

"A lot of work is being done to radically rethink the experience for our Vets and to make access to VA healthcare more convenient," says Evans. Looking to the future, Evans and the VA team are hard at work developing new connected health solutions, continuing to move care into patients' daily lives and routines whenever possible. As Evans sees it, the purpose of this and other initiatives is simple, "This is all about getting the patient's voice into healthcare."

In this chapter I've covered two examples that challenge the conventional wisdom that healthcare delivery can't and won't change—one from the point of view of disrupting the traditional system and one from the point of view of improving it. Walgreens gives us any number of examples of how we can offer services directly to consumers in this brave new world of twenty-first-century healthcare delivery. The VA offers a blueprint for healthcare providers on how to modernize their approach to the ancient art of medicine.

For businesses that wish to succeed in the new world of IoHT, two fundamental questions must be answered: Do you want to sell into the healthcare system as it exists? or Do you wish to compete with a system that is ripe for disruption?

7

Up Close and *Hyperpersonal*

"Apps can do so much more than we ever believed to be possible."

—Kamal Jethwani, MD, MPH, senior director,
Connected Health Innovation, Partners HealthCare

When we began creating the technical platforms for our connected health programs, we were laser-focused on figuring out how to get patient-generated data out of the home, into the cloud, securely into our database and our patients' electronic medical records. We naively thought that collecting objective data about each individual and sharing it with him or her in a classic feedback loop would prompt sustainable behavior change. Certainly, objective data are better than self-reported data—there is no hiding from those numbers. But as we learned, simply raising awareness is a relatively weak motivator; the novelty of having your health data displayed for you automatically, in real time, wears off pretty quickly. We gained these insights by constantly keeping in touch with our patients as we implemented various pilot programs over the years.

Patients tell us that they stay engaged with our chronic illness tracking programs largely because they know that someone in their doctor's office is watching the data. In fact, we showed early on that the more our practitioners log into the system to look at the dashboard view of these patient-generated vital signs, the better the patients do.

There are two factors at work here that tap into our desire to look good to others. First is social desirability bias, which I mentioned in Chapter 4—the idea that when our health data are presented in a social context we tend to "bring our A game" to impress our social networks. A variation on this is the Sentinel Effect—we behave differently when we know we're being watched. Patients want to please their doctor (and by extension, their doctor's staff). When they know that their doctor's staff are looking at these objective health data, most will instinctively pay more attention to all of their health-related tasks: exercise, diet, medication regimen, and so on. *You could say that our first phase of learning in building our tools was understanding the power of objective data to raise awareness and the second phase was the power of the Sentinel Effect.*

If you are building an engagement tool, particularly to improve the health of patients with chronic illness, and you build in these two principles, you will do pretty well at a population level. You will certainly do much better than a self-report system with no sense of someone watching. These design principles are second nature to us now, but we still find pockets of patients who won't engage. Leveraging the Sentinel Effect and the power of objective data is not enough to engage all comers. And if we want to bring healthcare costs under control and implement true population health, we need to have a goal of engaging *all* of these people.

The "last mile" of patient or consumer engagement is about personalization down to the individual level, or *hyperpersonalization*. This is a daunting problem, but we have some early evidence, as I will describe later, which makes me optimistic that we can solve this. I should also add that the vision of how to achieve this goal has some restrictions.

First, we can't simply add more staff—we'll never get healthcare costs under control if we just keep hiring people. The second restriction is we can't simply dump more work on our current staff. There are a multitude of studies that show loading healthcare workers with more tasks leads to critical errors and lapses in patient safety. There is only one way we can achieve success—we must automate some of our engagement processes. The third restriction is that our patients cannot feel neglected, bereft of human contact or cheated of time with their doctor. I've mentioned this before, but it bears mentioning again:

Patients will be turned off if they feel they are being subjected to a brittle, nonresponsive, mechanical form of interaction. You all know how frustrating it is when you call in to yet another automated voice response system and push keys to get through the logic tree so you can (sometimes) actually talk to a real person. As healthcare providers, we have to do much better. We know from past experience that it can be done well; I refer back to the story in Chapter 5 about Tim Bickmore's relational agents and how patients *preferred* the agent to a human being. *We can automate a great deal of motivational patient engagement, but we have to be very thoughtful about how we do that.*

This chapter is devoted to discussing where we are in this journey. At Partners we've moved on to our third phase of learning and have embarked on tackling a challenging piece of the puzzle: Improving our understanding of the human beings for whom we are designing personal health technologies and solutions. We think this will get us to that last mile of engagement.

WHO ARE YOU?

As mentioned above, our ultimate goal is to design a hyperpersonalized program for each individual that is as unique as the person who uses it; in theory, no two programs would be exactly alike because no two human beings are exactly alike. You may remember my Virtual Coach, Sam, from Chapter 1, who was not only able to anticipate my actions, but also provide me with precisely the right cues to keep me on track with my health goals. At times it seemed as if Sam knew me better than I knew myself—and that is precisely our goal. In all honesty, we're nowhere near there yet, but we have made some enormous strides in that direction in recent years.

To use a marketing analogy, remember back in the day when advertisers relied on zip codes as a primary means of market segmentation because they had little else to go on. A zip code told them something about your income and neighborhood, and what people "like you" were likely to respond to. Today zip codes seem primitive in contrast to having someone's entire online shopping history at our fingertips. It's no longer what people "like you" buy, we now know exactly what *you* have bought and we even know what products you've been looking at and what cues get you to click onto a website.

Healthcare, sadly, is pretty much back in the zip code era—with most clinicians reflexively segmenting patients on *clinical* grounds, which is a very broad measure. We adjust our treatment approach depending on a patient's laboratory numbers and other test results like their hemoglobin A1c (HbA1c), the clinical measure of blood sugar control for diabetes, ejection fraction for congestive heart failure, or systolic blood pressure for hypertension. In each of these cases, it's easy to categorize patients based on their physiologic parameters and prescribe treatment accordingly.

But this method of clinical segmentation sheds no insight into whether or not the person will take his medication as directed or make any of the other lifestyle changes that may have been recommended by his provider. It's not all that different from stuffing envelopes full of coupons into mailboxes without knowing what products are suitable for which households. And if it's important for marketers of consumer goods to understand their consumers better, it is even more critical for those of us who are selling health. That's where the next part of this journey takes us—to understanding human behavior.

BREAKING THE DESTRUCTIVE CYCLE

Any healthcare provider can attest to the fact that it's very difficult—if not impossible—for even the most intuitive practitioner to discern what's really going on in a patient's mind during a brief office visit. Furthermore, people often don't want to talk with their doctor about deeply rooted fears, or may not even fully understand the factors fueling these fears.

Figuring out why people do what they do is going to be critical if we want to move engagement to a truly meaningful level. We pretty much know how to prevent most chronic diseases and even know how to treat and reverse many conditions if they are caught early enough. What we don't yet fully understand is how to get people to do what's in their own best interest. It's worth pointing out here that I'm talking about that subset of chronic illnesses that are essentially silent as they attack your system.

There is another whole group of unfortunate individuals who have a chronic illness that causes constant discomfort (inflammatory bowel disease, fibromyalgia and migraine are just three examples). Pain is a great motivator and these individuals are often quite engaged in wanting to get well, but still frustrated by the lack of solutions healthcare has to offer them. Their psychology is totally different.

In order to break the cycle of destructive behaviors that are fueling the epidemic of lifestyle-related diseases, we need to understand why people engage in these behaviors in the first place. Why is it that so many patients don't take their medicine as prescribed? Why do people binge on food they know is bad for them? Why do people avoid exercise even though they know inactivity is unhealthy?

The reality is, even when you ask people *why* they do *what* they do, they often may not fully understand their own behavior. According to neuropsychologist Meghan Searl, there are countless people who may sincerely want to make a positive change—like eat a healthier diet or get more exercise—but are never able to follow through. Even with the best of intentions, something always happens to sabotage their efforts.

Searl explains that, "Basically, much of what happens in the mind is automatic—occurring outside of our conscious awareness—responding to our current situation out of a collection of mental habits and scripts that may have little to do with the actual situation." In other words, she says, "Our conscious minds make up stories about our behaviors. We might see ourselves engaging in a particularly unhealthy habit, like eating junk food, but we tell ourselves a story about why we *think* that's happening. These stories may have a ring of truth to them, but we don't fully acknowledge the extent to which these automatic habits are driving our behavior."

The root of these automatic behaviors can go back decades, often to childhood. We're not going to get too analytic here; suffice it to say, it's complicated. Searl acknowledges that these are difficult concepts for healthcare professionals to understand, let alone individuals struggling with trying to change their lifestyle habits. *Well-designed technology can play an important role in breaking through some of these barriers by raising awareness of what we're doing, if not why we're doing it.*

Searl goes on: "Awareness is a big key to making long-term sustainable change. But in addition to tracking behavior, which may be helpful to some people, we also need to figure out how to help people develop better coping skills for issues that are difficult and painful to think about. Sometimes we need more soul-searching or problem solving skills or emotional coaching in order to access that awareness, to allow that awareness to arise without just pushing it away."

GETTING TO THE "WHY"

Getting to the "why"—or learning as much as possible about what makes patients or consumers tick—is central to our research. Simply put, if we're going to create programs to change human behavior, we need to understand it better. It's no secret that consumer acceptance of health technologies has been spotty, often failing the people who need it the most. The recent industry-wide discussion (or obsession) with "patient engagement" is an acknowledgment of this failure, and the desire to do better.

One of the problems is that health technologies tend to be very generic. Basically, a device captures personal health data that is then displayed on an app or dashboard. Depending on the device or app, the individual may receive an encouraging message, something like, "You've only got 3,000 more steps to go to reach your daily goal." Or, "Don't forget to eat more salad today." There are lots of problems with this approach, which I'll get into later, but the primary downfall is that these messages really aren't personal. Sure, these prompts may be based on one or two data points collected about the person, but they also may be completely irrelevant to what's going on in that person's life at the moment.

The reality is, if we're going to sell health, we need to do a better job of learning about our consumer and we need to use that information to create just the right motivation at just the right time.

Smart marketers understand that making a strong connection to the *individual*—not just to the *market segment*—is an absolute requirement for selling to today's consumers. As observed in the 2015 Global Data-Driven Marketing Survey conducted by Teradata Corporation, "Among the myriad of eye-opening findings, one of the most notable is that having individualized insight is increasingly important to marketers." According to this report, 90%

of marketers say that making marketing individualized is a priority. And more to the point, "They want to move beyond segmentation to true one-to-one personalization in a real-time context."

If "one-to-one personalization in a real-time context" is a key factor in selling products and services, it is even more critical for selling health! As we know, the healthcare consumer is a tough customer. Many people don't know or acknowledge that they have a health problem, and even if they do, they may not be motivated to do what it takes to fix it. It often takes some convincing to move them to address a health issue or to create a mindset where they'll even consider making needed behavior changes.

Personalization is absolutely critical, but so is "in real-time context." Mobile technology enables us to get closer to our patient/consumer and to reach out to her with the right message at just the right moment when she needs us. Our research has shown that a well-timed text message that is relevant to an individual's frame of mind, as well as to what's happening in her life, is a powerful tool for behavior change. We have also found that it's far more challenging to create connected health solutions that reflect a deep understanding of what motivates each individual person, tapping into *why* someone does what he or she does.

ASK WHAT THEY WANT-WATCH WHAT THEY DO

Understanding the need to better connect to people as *individuals* has changed how we approach each project. We initially followed what I would call a traditional research model. That is, a primary investigator with an idea would pull together a team of other experts, design a program or device, build it and then give it to patients. Frequently, what seemed like a great idea in the abstract didn't work very well in real life with patients. Or, it might work for one small group of patients, but not for the majority, and we often found few if any patients would use a new device for more than a brief period.

After seeing that scenario repeat itself time and again, we rethought our product development process. Tim Hale of our team, whom I introduced in Chapter 4, describes it this way, "Today our approach is, 'Let's let the patients tell us what they want and need.' Before we build our prototypes, we do a lot more formative research. We ask lots of questions about patients' experiences of their illnesses and treatments, the barriers to care patients may be facing and what types of interventions and technology they think would be helpful. We work together with patients to create solutions to address their needs and get their input on prototypes to see whether or not they think our products will be useful to them. Now, it is an iterative process to figure out what will work. We also do a lot of observation of how people interact with technology to gain insights into needs that patients can't articulate."

Hale continues: "Along the way, we also learned that just because two patients have the same disease, they might not have anything in common beyond the same diagnosis. One patient can have a very different attitude toward managing his disease than another. That's why a generic, one-size-fits-all approach would be doomed to fail." For example, Hale says, "In the case of diabetes, there are all sorts of different scenarios within that patient population. Why are some people not taking their insulin? That's one group we need to address. Other individuals are taking their insulin but have difficulty maintaining tight control of their blood sugar and need to modify their diet and better track what they are eating. That's another group. Then there are people who might be able to control their diabetes and stop taking insulin if they could make and sustain changes to their lifestyle to lose weight and make healthier food choices. That's a different group and they need a different app or intervention strategy than each of the other two. We're beginning to create more customized apps that target one intervention within one subgroup of these medical conditions."

A MESSAGE AS POWERFUL AS A DRUG

Text2Move, Partners most ambitious effort to date, is considered by us to be the gold standard of what learning about your consumer means. Text2Move was not created to be about weight loss or dieting. The purpose of the project was to see whether highly personalized, targeted text messages, delivered at just the right moment, could boost activity levels among a fairly sedentary population of people with Type 2 diabetes.

It is well known that exercise is important for everyone, but is especially critical for people with diabetes in terms of helping them better manage their symptoms and avoid developing complications. So, it makes sense to prescribe exercise for everyone with diabetes. But getting people who are not in the "fit and fabulous" minority to engage in physical activity on a consistent basis is extremely challenging. We hoped that Text2Move would deliver the right "nudge" to get people started on a regular exercise program.

Text2Move turned out to be more successful than we ever could have imagined. This innovative, six-month behavioral modification program produced, on average, an impressive 1% drop in hemoglobin A1c (the clinical measure of blood sugar control). By established medical standards, a 1% decrease is considered significant and reduces the risk of heart attack by 14% and diabetes-related death by 21%. To put this in perspective, the usual drug treatment for this condition, metformin, gives on average a 0.5 gm drop in A1c, so our texting intervention was at least as powerful as an oral drug.

Let me share a bit about the thinking that helped to shape this program. From the beginning, we didn't want to create yet another pedometer-style walking app that provided generic feedback. Our goal was to delve a bit deeper into the psyche of our users and, more specifically, figure out the right "hook" that would resonate with each person. We wanted to go beyond simply collecting activity data and spitting back canned "inspirational" messages. Each message needed to feel as if it was crafted specifically for the person who was reading it.

We knew from experience that this was going to take some figuring out. The diabetic population we were targeting was hardly homogeneous. Some people knew that becoming more active would be helpful, but weren't ready to do anything about it. Others were eager to try something new and would embrace technology that would help them meet their goals. And then there were the people in-between, who were interested but needed some prodding to get going. How do you create a program that accommodates the needs of all these different types of people?

Our researchers and clinicians poured through the psychological literature on behavioral science and agreed that the app should be designed around the

Transtheoretical Model of Behavior Change, or what is popularly known as the "readiness concept." Developed in the 1990s by James O. Prochaska, PhD, and other researchers at the University of Rhode Island, the Transtheoretical Model identifies five stages of readiness to assess how willing someone is to make a health-related behavior change. These include "pre-contemplation," "contemplation," "preparation," "action" and "maintenance."

We understood the importance of approaching someone at the right time with the right message from our previous experience with patients. If someone isn't ready to hear what we have to say, that person will simply tune us out. We knew that assessing each person's readiness level ahead of time would give us an advantage in terms of making the program feel personal.

To further our understanding, we randomly selected 200 patients from Diabetes Connect, our web-based remote glucose-monitoring program that supports diabetes care between office visits. Each participant was asked to fill out a standard online questionnaire to assess his or her readiness level. Based on the answers, each participant was assigned a rating. Interestingly, we found that administering the questionnaire online was not only more efficient, but made it more likely that patients would actually finish it.

We also did some in-depth, face-to-face interviews to get a deeper understanding of what would motivate an individual to go out and take a walk. We asked questions like, "What would be the ideal conditions for you to take a walk?" The responses would run the gamut from, "I would take a walk on a sunny day before work as long as I didn't have an 8 a.m. meeting" to "I would only walk after work if it's not too cold or snowing." From these responses, we created a databank of 1,000 unique messages designed to reflect these different conditions and attitudes.

We then gave each study participant an activity tracker that tracked the number of steps that person walked daily. (We also gave trackers to a control group of diabetics who did not receive the text messages.) Over a six-month period, each participant would receive two messages each day, or a total of 180 texts over the duration of the study. One message reported the person's step count; the other message was a computer-generated message based on the person's behavior patterns and readiness scores.

Our learning algorithm took the dynamic data from the pedometer and determined whether the person had moved from one readiness stage to the next. Over the six-month study, we tracked each patient's changes in behavior to continually reassess his or her readiness level. This enabled us to create the impression of highly personalized messages written just for the recipient. For example, if the algorithm noticed that someone who was in the active phase and had been consistent about walking had suddenly gone off track, the message would reflect that. Instead of just telling him to take a walk, it would say, "Your activity declined since yesterday. Don't worry about it, just pick it back up again like you did on Monday."

Over time, the program began to know more about each person's behavior patterns and specifically what resonated with that individual. That helped us further personalize the person's messages. The more "it" learned about the person, the more targeted the messaging.

For instance, the algorithm noticed that one study participant would take a walk in the morning in bad weather, but in good weather, she would take her walk at night. As a result, it stopped sending her "get out and take a walk" messages on mornings when the weather was good and instead sent them at night. Another study subject took his walks around 2 a.m. every night. Our algorithm detected this and began sending out reminders at around 1 a.m. After the study, when we reviewed the data and saw the 2 a.m. messages, we immediately believed that it was an error (who would take a walk at that time of night?). But as it turned out, the patient was a shift worker who got off at 1 a.m. We (humans) never would have programmed a message to go out at 1 a.m., but the algorithm knew better.

In addition to producing a drop in A1c, our personalized messages appeared to produce a noticeable improvement in activity. For participants in the intervention group (the people who wore a pedometer and received daily text messages), the average daily step count was 1,300 to 1,400 steps more than the control group who wore a pedometer but did not receive text messages.

Again, it's important to note that Text2move is an entirely automated program. And that, in part, could be why it was so

successful. From this study, we learned that computer systems
could identify trends in a way that human eyes cannot.

Text2Move is not an app—it's a text messaging program. It was linked to the patient's medical information from their electronic medical records and from weather data retrieved from their mobile phone, but it did not have access to other features on the smartphone. We are now building on the technology of Text2Move to create even more personalized programs that leverage the technologies built into smartphones and that take advantage of social networking.

EMBEDDED IN YOUR LIFE

In the near future, we're going to have a lot more data about you. Right now, your smartphone, wearable devices and other technologies can provide a treasure trove of information about you that could be vital to helping you stay healthy. These technologies can track your location, where you inputted the data, if you logged onto Facebook or had a phone call before you did so. Think about how much more personalization will be possible with these data streams! If I know what you had for breakfast, how far you've walked, what your favorite song on Spotify is when you're at the gym, how many outbound messages you've sent your friends, how much time you spend on social media (and doing so many other things), I will be able to message you in such a personalized way that you'll be convinced that the software doing the messaging actually "knows you."

At some point in the not too distant future, our genome will be incorporated into our electronic medical records and that information will also be factored into creating hyperpersonalized programs. Telling someone to "Take a 30-minute walk because it's good for your heart" is not nearly as persuasive as telling someone, "Based on your genetics, taking a 30-minute walk today could reduce your risk of heart disease by 30% and substantially increase the odds that you will live past 85 in a healthy body." Or, instead of saying, "You gained two pounds this week, you need to watch your weight more closely," imagine how much more effective it would be to say, "If you don't watch your calorie intake at age 30, you are genetically predisposed to become obese by age 50." With these new tools, information that was once abstract can become very real.

So what are the takeaways for businesses from all this?

- Objectively collected information from wearables is good for raising awareness. This is useful for education and early engagement but generally not sustainable (unless the user is highly committed to a healthy lifestyle and thus probably not a sufferer of chronic illness). On the other hand, self-reported data is almost useless because of the intrusion of social desirability bias.

- Building some type of Sentinel Effect into product design will get you a long way (especially if combined with objective data collection). Depending on your starting point, this can lead to a very successful intervention if viewed at the population level. But this is an area where healthcare providers have an unfair advantage over others in the industry who desire to change health behaviors (payers, disease management companies, corporate wellness providers, for example). Because we have such a strong relationship with our patients, we can leverage the Sentinel Effect quite effectively in program design.

- The opportunity to automate health messaging around behavior change is vast. We can take some lessons from the advertising industry as it has made great strides in personalized presentation of ads. However, we also know that it is much easier to motivate people to make an impulse purchase than to adopt a healthy behavior, so there is still much to learn in this area. Those who are experts in machine learning and predictive analytics could partner with experts in the psychology of behavior change to make real inroads here. There is a clue in the contrasting stories of frustration with interactive customer service voice response (how *not* to design automated care) and Tim Bickmore's story, which I related in Chapter 5, about relational agent interactions that were preferred to human interactions.

- Finally, remember the anchoring tenets necessary for achieving this ambitious goal of automating care: We can't hire more staff, patients must feel cared for and providers can't feel overwhelmed with more work.

· · ·

YORN HEALTH: WHAT ARE THEY THINKING?

"Reputation now is not only based on the prestige of the staff or the waterfall in the lobby, it's the treatment. By that I mean it's not just how well you treat patients clinically, but how well you treat them as people."

—Brian McGoff, vice president, Yorn Health

The bathroom in her hospital room looked like it hadn't been cleaned in days; the nurse seemed brusque and disinterested; and when the wrong food tray arrived, it was the last straw. The 72-year-old heart patient decided to discharge herself from the hospital earlier than her doctor had recommended. Unfortunately, a few days later, she was back in the ER with new symptoms.

This is a hypothetical scenario, but one that happens more often than you would think, according to Brian McGoff. It's also precisely the type of poor outcome that Yorn—short for Your Opinion. Right Now.—was designed to prevent. Yorn is a real-time mobile platform that enables patients and authorized caregivers to provide feedback *in the moment* directly to healthcare institutions, providers and payers using secure Health Insurance Portability and Accountability Act (HIPAA)–compliant messaging and dashboards.

Utilizing what Yorn calls "experiential telemetry," the company integrates its patient-generated data with quantitative data from electronic health records, medical records, devices and other sources to create a profile of a patient's overall care experience. A patient's experiential profile can then be compared to profiles of similar patients with known outcomes to inform appropriate treatment and care plans. In other words, Yorn not only gives patients an opportunity to voice their concerns as a problem or question pops up, but provides hospitals with a new tool to better customize treatment and improve outcomes.

The mission to keep patients happy comes naturally to Yorn's founder and CEO Richard Rasansky, who has a background in the hospitality industry as well as technology. Among other ventures, Rasansky co-founded the highly acclaimed and innovative global hospitality company China Grill Management in New York City in the late 1980s.

Running a restaurant forces you to keep the needs of the consumer top of mind. If people don't like the way you're treating them, they'll take their business elsewhere. And bad word of mouth—like a string of bad reviews—can kill your business. Hospitals are finding out the hard way that the same rules may apply to them.

Unhappy patients are also voting with their feet. For example, McGoff notes that up to 2% of all admitted patients self-discharge before the recommended time. This is costly to the hospital in a number of ways. First and foremost, the same patient who "storms out" of the hospital could wind up back in the ER within a short amount of time, which (depending on the problem) could subject the hospital to a fine. And even if a patient stays but suffers in silence, as many do, an unhappy patient is not likely to refer family or friends to that hospital or even to that physician, which could be a significant loss in revenue. Not to mention the fact that disgruntled patients are more likely to give a hospital a poor rating in the Hospital Consumer Assessment of Healthcare Providers and Systems (HCAHPS) survey, a standardized, publicly reported survey of patients' perspectives of hospital care developed by the Centers for Medicare & Medicaid Services (CMS) and the Agency for Healthcare Research and Quality (AHRQ).

According to McGoff, "Often, by the time the hospital administrator gets to reading the discharge report, the real reason the patient left is never fully explained. If the hospital doesn't know a problem exists, it can't correct it. Even worse, patients who feel that they're not being listened to don't feel well cared for."

Instead of patients packing up and leaving—or allowing their anger to simmer—Yorn provides them (and designated caregivers) with a means to communicate in real-time with hospital personnel. Once the app is accessed from any mobile device, the easy-to-use platform allows the patient to communicate his thoughts or ask questions at any time, day or night, through postdischarge.

"The idea is it never gets turned off," McGoff explains. "Let's say you're coming in for a total hip or knee replacement. The minute you make your first appointment, you would get a text and an email that says, we (the hospital) care about you and your experience while you're here. At any time you want to provide us with feedback on that experience, tap here and let us know what you think." For example, if the patient finds the room untidy, or gets the wrong meal, she can send a message via Yorn, and the problem can be quickly resolved.

Yorn's initial healthcare client was the University of Pennsylvania Health System (Penn Medicine) for use throughout its inpatient and outpatient healthcare systems. The catalyst for this client relationship was based on the successful results of a three-month pilot program conducted by the Penn Medicine Center for Healthcare Innovation and the Department of Clinical Effectiveness and Quality Improvement, also located there. This pilot program resulted in increased patient satisfaction scores and higher quality ratings on performance.

Richard Rasansky believes that real-time feedback is transformational to improving overall performance. According to Rasanksy, traditional survey methods are designed to *avoid* listening to patients. They measure performance against preset standards—without direct, candid, detailed insight from the patient's point of view. Real-time feedback gives an active and participatory voice to patients when it matters most to them—and that interaction should be a significant part of the care process.

8

Try a Little Dopamine

In January 2015, researchers at the University of Missouri School of Journalism published a study that uncovered a new modern-day malady—iPhone separation anxiety. According to this study, students who were separated from their iPhones performed less well on cognitive tests, like solving simple word search puzzles, than when they had their iPhones close by. And, if the students were unable to answer their iPhones during these tests, "heart rate and blood pressure increased, self-reported feelings of anxiety and unpleasantness increased and self-reported extended self and cognition decreased. These findings suggest that negative psychological and physiological outcomes are associated with iPhone separation . . ."

The concept of iPhone separation anxiety piqued my interest because, for some time, my team and I have been exploring the phenomenon of smartphone addiction. We've been pondering why people become so attached to their smartphones that they quite literally can't keep their hands off them, yet have a "take it or leave attitude" when it comes to technology designed to improve their health. It's no secret that tens of thousands of personal health trackers wind up gathering dust and hundreds of thousands of health apps are abandoned within a month or so after they're downloaded. Yet, the opposite is true when it comes to smartphones—people can't seem to get enough of them.

According to a 2013 Kleiner Perkins industry report, we look at our smartphones about 150 times a day on average. Even when they're not ringing or buzzing, we check our phones for absolutely no reason other than we want to.

No wonder adjectives like "romance," "love affair"—even "addiction"—have been used to describe our strong attachment to smartphones!

I admit, this led to a bad case of "phone envy" on our part. We asked ourselves, "Why are smartphones so addictive, yet health trackers and apps so easy to forget?" And this led us to wonder: Can we create a health tech experience that would be as irresistible or "addictive" as a smartphone?

Many have talked about the transformational possibilities of mobile health. Always on and always connected, smartphones offer the opportunity to message you in-the-moment about health. These devices can also capture health-related information about you via the camera and connected sensors, and they have the ability to display relevant information in context. These technologies are exciting, but when it comes to health, they don't guarantee consumer engagement.

We are at a critical inflection point with health apps and devices. Consumer mobile app companies count downloads, but this is simply not a good enough measure of engagement when it comes to health. *We need to track and achieve sustained engagement with these tools to make a difference.* If you get disenchanted with your tracker and purchase a different one, both companies win. If you abandon them both due to disinterest, those who pay the bill for your healthcare costs may lose. This conundrum is magnified when we consider that the very group of individuals who can most benefit from health apps and trackers seem least interested in engaging with them at all.

I can understand why it is more appealing to go after the consumer wellness/fitness market than to take on the challenge of engaging those with chronic illnesses such as diabetes and hypertension. But in order to solve these vexing problems we need help. Elsewhere in the book I highlight various companies that are successfully moving the vision for the IoHT forward. However, when it comes to sustained engagement of folks with chronic illness to achieve measurable clinical results, the market is wide open. Yes, these are tough problems to solve, but look at it a different way. The wellness/fitness market is about 5% to 10% of consumers. Everyone is chasing that market now and, if you ask me, the market for trackers and apps feels a bit saturated.

On the other hand, of our $3 trillion in healthcare spending, 70% is related to lifestyle-influenced chronic illness. It is a much bigger market for anyone who can crack it.

This is why I came up with the catch phrase, *"Making health addictive."* What can we learn from people's obsession with their smartphones that could allow us to design our health trackers and apps more effectively?

A HEALTHY ADDICTION

Admittedly, the word addiction is laden with negative connotations. We associate addiction with harmful behaviors like drug abuse, alcohol dependency, smoking, gambling and, recently, even cravings for unhealthy sugary or high-fat foods. Addictive behaviors are often easily dismissed as lack of self-control—in other words, a sign of moral failure. In reality, addiction is a process in the brain caused by a substance or a behavior that results in a disruption in the brain's neurobiology.

When you consume an addictive substance, or engage in addictive behaviors, your brain is flooded with high amounts of dopamine, the "feel good" neurochemical. It creates a positive feedback loop, so that the more you gamble, for example, the more you will want to gamble. In fact, once the pattern of gambling and dopamine release is established, even *thinking* about gambling triggers the dopamine release—the biochemical explanation for cravings.

It turns out that smartphones are addictive, just not in quite the same way. CrackBerry jokes aside, smartphones tap into our brain's reward mechanisms, but to a lesser degree. Studies suggest that using smartphones produces a boost in dopamine, but not in the massive quantities associated with bad addictions. It's just enough of a spike to make us feel good without the euphoria associated with addiction.

The evolution of mobile apps has made the smartphone the proverbial Swiss Army knife of electronic devices. These devices were designed for bite-sized consumption of information and provide instant access to a seemingly endless stream of news, weather, financial reports, music, maps and much more. The information stream is constantly changing. Thus, whenever a smartphone user has some idle time, say waiting for an elevator, she will inevitably pull out her smartphone to check on what's new in the last five minutes. Each one of these logins leads to a small reward and that leads to the small release of dopamine setting up the "addiction" and craving.

The need to communicate is a profound human instinct and smartphones allow us to capture and share our lives, including photos and personal health data. Add to this the fact that the human brain craves novelty and new experiences, which smartphones can deliver in abundance.

It's not just that smartphones provide hours of content that is both entertaining and fun. The tasks we perform with the device meet certain basic human needs. "Smartphone activities appear to be aligned with motivational processes that are built into the human psyche," explains neuropsychologist Meghan Searl. "For example, most of us use our devices in part to fulfill our basic need for connection, whether it's through social media to find a date or texting to check up on family members. We often turn to devices to experience a sense of competence, like mastering a new word game or seeing that we have met our step count for the day. These technologies can also support our need for autonomy, from allowing us to create custom playlists of the music we enjoy to helping us manage our money with online banking."

Searl adds, "If smartphones were just machines that were always on, could do some cool things and had satisfying gestures built in, but didn't fulfill any of these motivational needs, I don't think that they would be addictive at all."

Smartphones have become such an integral part of our day-to-day lives that, to use the parlance of psychologists, they have become extensions of our "selves." We literally feel at a loss without them, or sometimes even engage in risky behaviors—like texting while driving—because we are unable to put them down.

In stark contrast to a smartphone, the pursuit of health offers little in the way of reward mechanisms. For most of the chronic illness–related health improvement behaviors, the reward is far in the future and abstract (like gaining a few days on your life expectancy or avoiding an event like a stroke). Thus, we ask these individuals to do something that requires effort, self-restraint or both, and the reward is only abstract. Health technology often asks people to do distasteful things, like draw blood to check glucose, monitor blood pressure (which can be anxiety provoking) or track food intake to monitor calories. That's why, instead of pursuing these activities, we seek to avoid them.

AWARENESS IS NOT ENOUGH

When we first conceived of connected health, the goal was simply to employ devices and create programs to easily capture data and feed it back to our patients/consumers. As I've said, this is called a feedback loop. Having this personal health information is helpful in order to establish awareness and to change people's mindset about their health. For instance, the National Weight Control Registry shows that people who weigh themselves more often tend to be better at keeping weight off than those who avoid the scale.

Even before fancy trackers came on the scene, a 2007 Stanford University study had analyzed 20 studies on using pedometers. The researchers found that, on average, pedometer wearers walked an additional 2,000 steps a day compared to when they were not wearing pedometers. The studies that were the basis of the article, which was published in *The Journal of the American Medical Association,* followed patients for an average of 18 weeks, but not long term. As the study's authors concluded, "The results suggest that the use of a pedometer is associated with significant increases in physical activity and significant decreases in body mass index and blood pressure. Whether these changes are durable over the long term is undetermined."

The challenge, we found, with feedback loops alone is that their ability to capture your attention and motivate you decays over time. In many cases, once the newness has worn off, people forget about these signals.

Health-tech developers need to do a great deal more than just spit back data to create a patient/consumer health experience that is as compelling, sticky and, yes, as addictive as a smartphone. I am not suggesting that we turn individuals into "addicts" whose brains have been hijacked by out-of-whack neurobiology. Making health addictive is really about harnessing the power of mobile devices, particularly smartphones, and using it to "sell" health. If people are already mesmerized by their smartphones, checking them 150 times daily, doesn't it make sense to put a personalized, relevant, motivational and unobtrusive message in front of them some of the time? It seems a natural evolution for health tech to exploit these opportunities.

At Partners we are developing the next generation of health technologies, which will incorporate some of the key features that make popular technologies "sticky" and that are currently lacking in the typical health experience. Although I would be the first to say that we haven't come up with all the answers yet (nobody has) we have made some real progress on this front. We've learned that what ultimately works is simple design combined with the right, highly personalized motivational strategies that resonate with each individual at the right moment, just when he or she needs it. As a result, we design our platforms around incorporating as many "reward" features into our connected health programs as we can, as well as subconscious triggers that keep people on track. Our team has spent a great deal of time researching, thinking, talking about and analyzing the addictive qualities of smartphones that could be used to create more appealing health technologies to help capture the interest and imagination of our patients. From our research, we've come up with three basic strategies, and three tactics, that we believe will not just connect people to their data, but also connect them to their health on a deeper level.

The three strategies are: (1) Make It about Life; (2) Make It Personal; and (3) Reinforce Social Connections.

The three tactics are: (1) Employ Subliminal Messaging; (2) Use Unpredictable Rewards; and (3) Use the Sentinel Effect.

I describe a bit about each below.

Strategy 1: Make It about Life

When a patient goes to the doctor, she is typically handed a clipboard with a form asking her to list her personal medical history, family medical history and any medications that she is taking. True, this is important information, but it's lacking what may be the most critical factors in getting her to adhere to the doctor's advice: What are her goals and aspirations? What does being healthy enable her to do that she couldn't do (or can't do) otherwise?

My point is, simply telling patients that high blood pressure increases their risk of having a heart attack or stroke is in all likelihood not going to be an effective method to get them to take their medication as prescribed, engage in more exercise, or do any of the things that would help control the condition. Likewise, having patronizing conversations with folks—threatening them with worsening chronic illness if they do not comply with their treatment plans—is really old school and largely ineffective. People tend to tune out scary news, especially when it's related to their health. What we really need to do is get inside a patient's head to learn about her goals and aspirations, and most of all, connect them to her health.

Perhaps that patient has been dreaming about going to Paris, but is worried that she won't have enough stamina to take the trip. Or maybe she's newly single and wants to look (and feel) more attractive so she can reenter the dating scene or look better in a bathing suit next summer. The trick seems to be making the message and the payoff less clinical, less technical, less abstract and more aspirational. ("I want to be less winded when I walk around on vacation." Or, "I want live long enough to enjoy my grandchildren.").

One of the best examples of the Make It about Life strategy is the day-in-the-life promotional video produced by Twine, the company I mentioned in Chapter 5. Twine produces a collaborative care platform that enables a health coach to manage patients with chronic illnesses like hypertension via text messaging. The video kicks off with Tony, an automobile mechanic, sitting down with Laura, his coach, to make a plan, which includes medication to lower his blood pressure. But the story line focuses on the relationship between Tony and his young granddaughter, Ellie. Tony calls Ellie to tell her he has to work late because he has to go to the doctor in the afternoon to deal with a medication problem and therefore can't visit her that evening. Ellie sounds so disappointed that Tony calls his Twine coach to see if he can reschedule the doctor's appointment. Much to his delight, the coach is able to contact the doctor to make the medication adjustment so that Tony can skip the appointment altogether and not have to make up that time at work. The video ends with Tony helping his granddaughter learn how to ride her new two-wheeler bike that evening. Any prospective patient watching that video could easily make the connection that using Twine would make his life easier and that better managing his condition would keep him healthy so that he could do the things that he loved to do. It's a pretty compelling message.

Effectively implementing the Make It about Life strategy will require a couple of important changes. One is to change medical school curricula to teach students about patients' mindsets regarding acute illness versus chronic disease management and how to implement effective behavior change programs. The second is to learn as much as we can about each individual in order to identify his or her personal, relevant aspirational goals. (This is also about getting to the "why," or finding the underlying motivation for behavior change that I talked about in the last chapter.) Here again, the smartphone comes into play, becoming both a data-rich environment and a data conduit to enable analytic systems to learn enough about you to help make those behavior change messages relevant.

Strategy 2: Make It Personal

Picture this: You live in a big city high-rise, you don't own a country home, you have absolutely no interest in growing things nor the place to do so even if you wanted to. You have never read a book about gardening or agriculture, or searched a gardening website. Yet, when you click onto Amazon, you are greeted with an entire page of offers for books on gardening and products like hoes, rakes and fertilizer. This would strike you as extremely odd because we expect a different experience from Amazon and, of course, this didn't actually happen. I'm using this unlikely scenario to make a point. When we log onto Amazon, our home page is filled with a curated selection of offerings based on previous shopping and searching behavior. Each homepage is highly individualized because, in all probability, no two people do exactly the same thing. The user feels that Amazon has made a real effort to "know" him and that the retailer is speaking directly to him. Health messaging should have the same hyperpersonalized approach. We should get the same "they really know me" feeling with each message and interaction.

In terms of personalization, mobile health has been slow to adapt. Simply telling someone that she should walk 5,000 more steps today or eat a salad for lunch is not very personal. It could apply to countless numbers of people. Telling someone that she should walk 5,000 steps to prepare for her trip to Paris is a different story. It feels personal. Adding links to special walking tours of Paris along with the text is both personal *and* aspirational. You get the idea. The more you can fine tune the message, the more it will feel like it's "just for me."

We can learn a great deal from smart marketers like Amazon and the advertising industry who are leading the way. The main reason newspapers and magazines are on life support these days is because it's virtually impossible to target print ads beyond simple variables such as zip code or rough income level. Web search and e-commerce have given advertisers a whole new level of personalization to target their messaging. The main technology at work here is "cookies," tiny pieces of code that advertisers embed in your browser to track your browsing habits when you log on to various websites. So, when you're researching new cars on the web and visit car dealer and manufacturer websites, you leave a cookie trail. That's why you're likely to see advertising from your local car dealer or promotions for the latest lease offer pop up in your Facebook or other social media pages. They know you are interested and are now able to zoom right in.

With this data, advertisers then build a profile of your browsing behaviors and compare you to other profiles, and the software predicts your interests based on those most like you. This is how recommendation engines for Amazon, Netflix and Apple work. When they get it right, it feels somewhere between eerie and pleasing. If you're not thinking too hard, you'll go with pleasing as in, "Wow, that is exactly what I was looking for." (I routinely marvel at how quickly Google predicts what I'm searching for as I type.) But if you think about it, you may also feel that "it's a bit creepy," realizing that some database in the cloud knows that much about you. And the technology keeps getting better. New technologies such as clickstream—defined by Wikipedia as "the recording of the parts of the screen a computer user clicks on while web browsing or using another software application"—are guaranteed to make the experience even more personal. Of course, all this is coming to your smartphone too.

We know that the advantages of personalized messaging also apply to healthcare as well. Folks who have enrolled in our mobile health programs for chronic illness management have told us that they stay engaged when the messages are personalized. We see this over and over again.

In Chapter 7, I described the Text2Move study we conducted to help people better manage their diabetes by increasing their activity levels. The text messages were programmed to take into account the subject's motivational state, activity level and the context of his or her neighborhood, all collected passively via sensors or by asking the person a few simple questions. We were blown away by the positive results, which I repeat here because they were so remarkable: Patients receiving automated, personalized messages walked, on average, 1,400 more steps daily than those who were simply tracking their steps. Over six months, those 1,400 steps translated into a 1% drop in hemoglobin A1c. This is an impressive result that I doubt we could have achieved if all we did was threaten the patient with chilling descriptions of life-changing complications of diabetes and sent them home.

So imagine a world where we are collecting information such as your activity level, GPS location and mobile purchasing data along with doing natural language processing analysis of your outgoing messages (tweets, texts, emails, and so on) to build your unique health-related profile. This will enable us to send you highly customized, personalized, relevant messages some of the times you check your phone (which, as noted earlier, can be up to 150 times per day).

Some of our health messages will be so subtle you may not even notice them. Some will be welcome and none of them will be annoying—*if we do it right.* By right I mean, we really must get to know and understand the consumer/patient and tailor our messaging accordingly. This is where we may see a blend of advertising and health messaging. On the one hand, those of us with the goal of changing health-related behaviors can learn a tremendous amount from those who design compelling ads. Also, there are any number of healthy purchases you might make in your quest to improve your health. Why not offer those businesses the opportunity to participate in the experience of making health addictive by integrating them into our apps?

Strategy 3: Reinforce Social Connections

There are many motivational tools showing up in products on the market these days—incentives, games and coaching to name a few. But those with a social component tend to have a greater impact. While not universal, the desire for affiliation runs deep and none of us wants to appear unhealthy to our friends or family. Social networks effectively increase accountability and adherence to care. And wellness plans and mobile phones make social interactions that much more convenient. Sharing health information in a social context illustrates the two powerful psychological phenomena I mentioned earlier: social desirability bias and the closely related Sentinel Effect. Both of these constructs remind us how powerful the effect of being watched is.

When we reveal certain aspects of our lives, we are more likely to want to emphasize the positive and minimize the negative. This is what leads to the criticism that Facebook pages are not a reflection of reality but of the reality we'd like. Likewise, when it comes to our health, we often go out of our way to emphasize—and might tend to overestimate—the positive, if left to our own devices. When reporting is anchored by an objective data source, such as an activity tracker or a blood pressure monitor, we realize that we can't select only the data we like. As a result, we compensate by improving the behaviors that are reflected in those objective data.

In fact, according to a recent Harris Interactive survey conducted on behalf of Wellocracy, our latest project to reach consumers with information and guidance on health tracking, the majority of Americans (68%) report that encouragement from family and friends is important for them in achieving health goals.

The Sentinel Effect is a more extreme idea, illustrating how people respond when they know they are being observed and evaluated. If the evaluator is your doctor, the tendency to want to improve health behavior goes up dramatically (for more on this, see Tactic 3, below).

These days, almost every mobile experience has the "share" option as an integrated component. As we think about making health addictive, and about how we can slip unobtrusive, personalized, motivational messages into your life as you constantly check your mobile device, making the experience social will have a big impact on adherence and success.

We have to make the experience so compelling, however, that you will want to share it with others. That's where the tactics come in.

Tactic 1: Employ Subliminal Messaging

The term "subliminal messaging" has its roots in the advertising industry. Social commentator and author Vance Packard first alerted people to this practice in his 1957 bestseller, *The Hidden Persuaders*. When I was a teenager, I remember stories about psychological experiments in which advertisers would splice still frames of product images or messages into unrelated film clips. Watching the film, you'd never actually see those images or messages, but they would subliminally imprint on your mind and influence your behavior. Another common use of the term refers to subtle visualizations in various advertising imaging that allegedly speak to the subconscious. A Google search will show you many examples, most with some sort of sexual double entendre.

The assumption is that subliminal messaging is evil because it gets us to part with our money for things that we may not really want or need. In other words, it tricks us into doing things that are not to our benefit. But suppose we hijack this powerful tool for the good? Instead of using subliminal messaging to get people to buy stuff, we use this tactic to motivate healthy behavior. While getting someone's attention with a colorful, catchy, fun, attractive or useful message of some sort, you'd slip in a health-related message. This tactic is an implementation tool for Strategy 1, Make It About Life. I have two examples to illustrate this tactic when applied to healthcare.

My favorite example of this phenomenon is the terrifically successful truth campaign for the American Legacy Foundation. They have employed every trendy teen movement you can think of—from texting and social media to concerts and online voting—all in the name of educating teens about how the tobacco industry manipulates its products. It's a fascinating approach. There is no admonishment about using tobacco per se, only lots of fun ways to bring teens into the conversation about how bad tobacco is for them. Imagine if every other time you checked your phone, an unobtrusive brief message appeared on *your* health issue and how to improve it.

The second example is from our own work at Partners. It involves a study we did a while back to test the impact of text messaging on sunscreen adherence. The headline that came out from the study was that a daily text message reminder was a powerful motivator of adherence (about 60% of the time compared to about 10% in a control group). What is even more relevant was the design of the messages. Each morning, our participants received a text message with the weather report and, secondarily, a reminder to apply sunscreen. In exit interviews, the most interesting thing study participants told us was that the thing that kept them coming back to read the text messages was the weather report. They didn't really pay attention to the sunscreen adherence message. They didn't object to it, but it didn't really strike them either. Yet, these study subjects were motivated to apply sunscreen about 60% of the time. That's pretty good adherence rate for a "forgotten" message!

I think you see where this is going. By designing health-related messages to appear within something that is funny, inspiring or just plain useful, it seems we can have a greater impact than messages that threaten, scold or embarrass an individual. I'm talking about the type of messaging that has, over the years, led so many of my dermatology patients to say to me, "Please don't yell at me because I got a sunburn." I confess, I never yell at patients, but the feedback is that we need to message better.

I saw a great quote recently, claiming that advertising is moving from the Mad Men generation to the Dr. Spock generation—from billboards and print ads to personalized, contextual, highly segmented messages based on our most recent digital behavior. This is where we need to go with health messaging—slipping these messages in front of you while you're indulging in that "oh so delicious" activity of checking your phone.

Tactic 2: Use Unpredictable Rewards

The concept of unpredictable rewards brings us closer still to the vision of what *making health addictive* might look like on your mobile device. This tactic is what the mobile industry has capitalized on to get you to check your device 150 times a day. Now, we just need to corral the power mobile devices have to call your attention to relevant, personalized health messages and in doing so change your behavior for the better.

This tool for behavior change is not new. In 1948, when B.F. Skinner did his famous operant conditioning experiments, he measured salivation in response to presenting a food pellet to a rat. In the background, he also rang a bell when the food pellet was presented. After a while, he observed that the rat would salivate when the bell rang, whether the food pellet dropped or not. The response was even stronger, however, when the food pellet was presented randomly. This observation was the beginning of the science of variable rewards.

Advertisers use this concept often, as they know how effective it is. One recent noteworthy example comes from the company Uber. Undoubtedly you have heard of Uber. They've turned the frustrating process of flagging a taxi upside down and in the process created a much more pleasant cab experience for the customer. Recently, the company did something else to increase engagement. Every now and then, when you open the Uber app, you will see an offer for something completely unrelated to getting a ride. It might be a discount on flowers or show tickets. They do this randomly and even though it's not part of their core business, they have demonstrated that people open the app more often knowing that this unpredictable reward might be there.

Tactic 3: Use the Sentinel Effect

One of my favorite quotes comes from a former patient who participated in our Connected Cardiac Care program, Partners' heart failure telemonitoring program. "There's a sense of security in knowing that people who are medically trained are looking after me. If I miss something, they'll pick it up," he said, and with a laugh added, "I have to be truthful with them, I can't fudge it [when talking about my eating behaviors] because I can't eat fudge!"

As I've already said, the Sentinel Effect is the tendency for human performance to improve when people are aware that their behavior is being evaluated. This is similar to the Hawthorne Effect, or behavior change as a result of being observed but not evaluated. Both are useful tools in the context of connected health. I've emphasized the Sentinel Effect because, in our experience, patients significantly increase their adherence to a variety of healthy behaviors when they know that their physician (or her agent) is watching. If the same programs were based on self-reported data from patients keeping a written diary, for example, we'd have much weaker outcomes. Patients would report those data that make them look healthy and ignore those that do not. As our patient noted, with remote monitoring, he couldn't "fudge" his data.

Our remote monitoring program for heart failure is designed to teach patients how to better manage their conditions with the goal of reducing hospitalizations. Heart "failure" is a condition in which the heart can't pump enough blood to meet the body's needs; it is the leading cause of hospitalization for people over age 65. Symptoms include sudden weight gain (due to fluid build-up, often from dietary sodium intake), as well as difficulty breathing and swelling of the extremities. With our remote monitoring program, each morning patients take their blood pressure, pulse and weight. In addition, patients answer symptom questions on a small touch-screen computer and transmit the data to Partners HealthCare at Home. A telemonitoring nurse reviews the data and, when readings are outside established parameters, initiates appropriate intervention. This includes a call to the patient to check on his or her condition and, when necessary, coordination with the patient's physicians.

We've learned a lot about the value of the Sentinel Effect from talking to patients in our home monitoring programs, who tell us they are diligent about sticking to a program because their doctor or nurse is watching. The thought of having an authority figure look in on your life is a really powerful tool that can be used to effectively promote good health through mobility.

In another program, we asked patients with diabetes to upload their blood glucose readings and gave them access to tables and graphs of their data. What we found is that patients' diabetic control, as measured by HbA1c, improved based on how many times the practice nurse logged on to the system. Patients told us that they would only upload their readings if they got the signal that it was useful to their doctor in providing their care. The proxy for this was the practice nurse calling them to talk about their data. Once again, they confessed they were more attuned to their illness when they knew they were being watched.

As healthcare providers, in the context of taking on more risk for clinical outcomes, the Sentinel Effect may be our biggest asset. Certainly, our relationships with our patients are stronger and more meaningful than relationships with health plans or pharmaceutical companies. It is somewhat sad, however, that both the heart failure and diabetes patients only engaged when they felt their doctor (or doctor's agent) was watching. It tells us that many people with chronic illnesses are content to delegate their care decisions to someone else. You can argue that we healthcare providers have fostered that passive approach, but whatever the origin, we need to move beyond it. As I see it, we have two choices: Either convince people they can manage these illnesses on their own most of the time and reward them for it *or* build an authoritative coaching voice into our messaging tools. In the short term, we probably need to do both.

Currently, we're contemplating whether we actually need a nurse or doctor as the "sentinel." For these algorithmic conditions, like uncontrolled hypertension, could we employ software to do the monitoring rather than having a doctor or nurse monitor the patient data? But would patients be as responsive and diligent managing their own health? Early results suggest this is possible, but research is ongoing.

REAL LIFE EXAMPLES

Are there examples of people putting these strategies and tactics into action to achieve sustained change in health behavior? I can't think of any in the healthcare space who are doing it . . . yet. So, as I wrap this chapter up, I'm forced to go to nonhealthcare examples to suggest how it might look if we put it all together.

The first example is Facebook Home. This now-defunct app was launched a couple of years ago for folks with an Android phone, giving them the opportunity to make Facebook their home screen. Whenever they opened their phone, they got whatever Facebook had to offer before they went on to their other phone-related tasks. This experiment was not successful and I can only conjecture that's because people felt it was too invasive. But imagine if your health plan offered you the opportunity to download an app that, each time you opened your phone, greeted you with a health plan–sponsored, health-related message tailored just for you. This could be subtle and nonintrusive. My hunch is that if it was highly personalized and relevant to everyday life, *and you got a guaranteed lower premium for engaging with such an app*, people might go for it. This idea combines Strategies 1 and 2 (Make It About Life and Make It Personal), above, and could include all three of the Tactics I covered, depending on how the messages were designed.

The second example is from Google and its app called Field Trip. This app uses the GPS on your phone and is location-aware. If you turn it on in downtown Boston (where I work and walk around), the phone will vibrate or play a sound anytime you walk by an historic site. You pull out your phone and you can read all kinds of content about that site. Imagine if "the system" knew your weight, vital signs, glucose level, activity level, sleep patterns and what you had for breakfast (all of these are now achievable). When you head out for lunch, your phone could help steer you to healthy choices that would fit into your life goals. This example also uses Strategies 1 and 2 and possibly all three Tactics, depending on how the messages are designed.

It is not hyperbolic to say again, *we're at an inflection point in using mobile tools to achieve sustained health behavior change.* Those companies that are able to design life-relevant, personal and social apps that use subliminal messaging, unpredictable rewards and an authoritative voice in their message design— *especially when combined with some sort of objective data feed from a tracker or wearable*—stand the best chance of achieving meaningful results.

What are the takeaways for businesses?

Remember, this chapter is about product design and focusing on what motivates people to engage, not what we've traditionally focused on in our medical view of illness:

- Design products that engage enough with consumers to help them craft health goals that are relevant to their life.

- Take a page from the advertising industry and create products that can learn about users, morph in real time and personalize both interfaces as well as messages.
- Employ social networking; it's one of the most powerful technological tools of the twenty-first century. By carefully building this functionality into products, combined with the personalization concept discussed above, you can offer competition to those who crave it, companionship to the lonely and the opportunity to achieve goals as a team.
- Embellish these three strategies with the tactics I've outlined in this chapter. Subliminal messaging enables you to offer a very compelling message and slip your health message in almost as an afterthought.
- Make unpredictable rewards an important part of sustained engagement. The human brain craves newness and this psychological trick provides just enough novelty to keep people coming back.
- Work the Sentinel Effect, the Hawthorne Effect and social desirability bias into product design. They are all subservient to the strategy of harnessing social connection, but they can be powerful motivators.

There is great opportunity here. Today's products are almost all unidimensional in this regard. One company offers a social solution to improve employee health. Another offers a tracker and team-based competitions. They all improve engagement double digits over baseline. Think about what a product could do that was life-relevant, personalized and knew exactly how to motivate an individual over time.

9

Making Data Actionable

"We think of it as offering a new microscope that provides a much richer picture of how people are doing outside of the clinic or hospital. And the information that you leave in your wake—your digital exhaust—can actually be used to infer your health state in a more objective and richer way than was ever before possible."

—KARAN SINGH, CO-FOUNDER, GINGER.IO

Big Data. Predictive analytics. Machine learning. These are the hot and hip buzzwords that are being bandied about as the cure for all of healthcare's ills and the incubators for the next generation of billionaires. And while there are business opportunities in many areas here, it's important to note that our understanding of how to use analytics in healthcare is comparable to the discovery of fire by our ancestors. It's a transformation tool, but we have much to learn before we can maximize its value.

The burning question is: How do we put analytics to work in healthcare? There is no simple answer, but the following explanation may help clarify how these new tools could significantly impact the way we practice medicine in the decades to come.

Imagine that you are in charge of getting 1,000 people to do a certain task. Based on earlier studies of the population, the group appears to complete the task about 10% of the time: Your job is to push that number up as high as possible and the stakes are high. You get paid $500,000 for every individual who completes the task, but you lose $750,000 for each one you fail to convert.

Since this is a visually oriented task, you start by trying it yourself and notice that if you put a green filter over your eyes, you can see the end point much more clearly. Immediately, you distribute green-tinted glasses to all 1,000 people. Let's say 50% (way more than the 10% who are already completing it without your intervention) put the glasses on and finish the task. That is a great result right? The trouble is, due to your financial agreement, you will just break even with this result. You scratch your head. It was so clear to you that when you put the green-tinted glasses on you could complete the task, but why didn't it work for everyone? You study the remaining 40% and find that 10% lost the glasses before putting them on because they were distracted; another 10% refused to put them on because they were paranoid and they thought that you were trying to control them; 10% did not hear you when you mentioned that wearing the glasses was required to complete the task; and the final 10% were red/green colorblind, so wearing the glasses gave them no insight.

ORDER FROM CHAOS

This example is a bit like the state of population health and analytics in healthcare today. The first thing it illustrates is that if order is your goal and you start with chaos, any bit of order will seem like a success. There are countless examples of chronic illness management interventions and corporate wellness programs that achieve about 40% to 60% engagement across the sample. For most of the health behaviors we want to promote, baseline adoption is about 10%. Forty percent looks good right? But what about the remaining 60%? If you look at it that way, the intervention is a failure.

Congestive heart failure is a disease we've talked about quite a bit in this book. It leads to increasing numbers of hospitalizations over time, as the patient's heart loses strength. Medicare is now asking hospitals to pay for some of these admissions, if they are within 30 days of a previous discharge. All of a sudden preventing readmissions for CHF patients is in vogue and there are some standard things that we do to monitor patients more closely. We can have a nurse call them or even send a nurse to their homes postdischarge. We can bring them in for outpatient follow-ups soon after discharge and monitor their vital signs with technology. We can give them technology to remind them to take their medications. All of these work for *some* of the patients *some* of the time. But like the visual task example, we don't want to rejoice at getting a 40% success rate because the other 60% are costing us money (and the quality of care is not great either).

The challenge for data science and analytics is to help us fine-tune our interventions so that we get as close to a 100% success rate as possible. Faced with changing payment models and pressure to improve outcomes and cut costs, payers and providers are now turning to predictive analytics to better manage and understand patient populations. The goal is to identify patterns of behavior that could indicate potential problems down the road and intervene earlier, when it might still make a positive difference in health outcomes. Companies like IBM, Optum, Oracle, Truven Health Analytics, SAS Institute, LexisNexis Risk Solutions, Inovalon, iHealth Analytics, Cerner, Ginger.io and Predilytics, to name a few, are part of the growing healthcare analytics market that is projected to be valued at $21.4 billion by 2020. So far, "descriptive analytics," a basic summation of data, represents the largest share of the market. The term means that your data can be analyzed and the attributes described. This clearly has limitations and, according to MarketsandMarkets, a global market research and consulting company, "predictive analytics and prescriptive analytics are the highest growing areas during the forecast period."

Predictive analytics takes it a step further. If you go back to our visual task example, predictive analytics might have identified that some percent of the population was color-blind and therefore would not respond to the green glasses intervention. The other ubiquitous example of predictive analytics enters our lives most days if we order from Amazon, watch Netflix or listen to Pandora. All of these companies have become expert at filling in the blanks on the following sentence: Others like Joe did [blank], therefore we can predict that Joe will also do [blank]. If you use your imagination a bit, you'll conclude that this approach is probably not going to get us to the end zone in health behavior change.

If Netflix recommends a movie that I think is a miss for me, I can move on, but if an algorithm recommends a health behavior for me and the conditions are not just right, I'll probably be annoyed or offended, leave and not come back. The goal, then, is to take predictive analytics to another level and get to know you so well, we can predict what you will do uniquely rather than what "folks like you" would do. As stated earlier, we're just starting to think about the implications of this in healthcare.

THE POINT OF DATA

Financial services companies and retailers have long recognized that the "data exhaust" people leave behind in their everyday lives is a valuable source of information to be mined, analyzed and put to good use (more on that later in this chapter). And, healthcare is finally catching up. The hot commodity is an individual's "data points," the digital footprint created whenever a person uses a credit card or customer loyalty card, makes a deposit or withdrawal from an ATM, drives through a tollbooth, books a vacation online, buys a book from Amazon, visits a website, downloads an app, renews a driver's license, wears a health tracker, or communicates via social media. In essence, data points can be produced whenever a person does *anything* that is digitized, stored in the cloud and accessed by organizations interested in following behavior patterns. Combining nonclinical data with clinical data from EMRs, for example, can be a powerful tool in terms of predicting which patients are headed for trouble.

It is worth mentioning how groundbreaking this approach is in healthcare. Let's return to our CHF example. As clinicians, we're taught to segment populations on one dimension only—clinical. In the case of CHF, the number is called an ejection fraction, which is a numeric measure of how strong the heart muscle is. Over the years, I've heard folks say things like, "We chose to use this intervention only on patients with an ejection fraction less than 25%." We're now learning that that number alone is not sufficient. We should also be looking at the mental health dimension, the health literacy dimension, and the technology readiness dimension to name a few in a long list of possibilities.

The data dust we leave behind is another dimension that can help fill the gaps in the story. Some of you may have seen the television commercial for

Bayer aspirin showing a middle-aged man reading an ominous note that was left on the windshield of his car that says, "Your heart attack will happen tonight." A somber voiceover quickly explains, "David's heart attack didn't come with a warning. . . ."

When I saw the ad, it occurred to me that there may have been warnings along the way that nobody captured. Suppose David, our heart attack victim, was taking medications for both high blood pressure and high cholesterol, and was on a diet and exercise program to lose weight and improve his cardiac health. And suppose he had a history of not being vigilant about taking his medications. And suppose several months before his heart attack, he stopped working out at the gym, was eating more take-out food (which he conveniently ordered online) and was skipping payments on his credit cards, although he had always paid on time. While some of this information may not be directly related to his health, any of these factors could be a red flag that something in David's life was amiss. Perhaps he was under a great deal of stress at work, leaving him little personal time to take care of himself and his finances, or perhaps he wasn't feeling well and lacked the energy and motivation to maintain his healthy routine.

If these behavior changes had been spotted early enough, it might have been possible to intervene, improving his general health and stress level and lessening the chance of an adverse cardiac event. And just imagine if David had been wearing an activity tracker and participating in a program to self-monitor his blood pressure and weight, and sharing that information with his provider. It's hard to believe that somewhere along the line, the change in his health status wouldn't have been detected and some sort of intervention prescribed.

CHANGING THE CONVERSATION ABOUT HEALTH

How does connected health change the conversation about health analytics? Connected health is about collecting data (*objective* data as much as possible rather than *self-reported* data) from patients outside of medical settings to provide a more realistic view of their health status in real life. Combined with non-clinical data—the everyday stuff that doesn't appear to have anything directly to do with health—this helps put the clinical and passively collected data into the context of someone's life. Hence, the Internet of *Healthy* Things—personal health trackers, GPS in smartphones and watches, embedded sensors in clothing and electronics and social media activity—can provide additional data sources relevant to improving health and wellness.

The richness of the data we can collect is breathtaking and it puts the notion of predictive analytics at the individual level in sight. A good example is in the realm of medication adherence. The state of the art is to look at various pharmacy claims to ascertain if an individual has taken medication as prescribed.

I take a statin daily and someone analyzing data from my insurer or my pharmacy would conclude that I am adherent because I've been picking up my refills every 90 days since the drug was prescribed. Refill rates and pharmacy claims can give us a crude measure of whether someone is taking a medication, but offer no insight into *why* that person is not taking it. They offer no insight into whether I'm taking my meds on time and at the right time of day. And if I don't take a medication, is it because I forgot, I'm confused or I can't afford it? There are now more than 100 companies offering technologies that track medication adherence at the individual pill or injection level. These technologies can give us a granular view of medication adherence and allow us to infer patterns of behavior leading to nonadherence.

Changes in behavior patterns, clinical data from an EMR, and tools used by marketers to monitor such things as shopping preferences, can provide a much more detailed portrait of an individual than can be gleaned from a once- or twice-a-year visit to the doctor.

Nick van Goor, PhD, head of Data Science at Honeywell Connected Homes (and formerly with Teradata), observes that looking at what people do in their everyday lives can provide a window into their heath behaviors. "There's the direct evidence that relates to monitoring connected things; what you do with your phone, where you go during the day, that kind of stuff, that's *direct data*," Van Goor explains. "But there's also a lot of *inferential* data that you can get about people's behaviors that are widely used in the marketing space. For example, I did a project around 15 years ago where we looked at credit card data. Looking back three years, if I know everywhere someone has shopped over that period of time, it tells me a great deal about a person. Anything that you buy online—even the websites you visit—is recorded and that reflects pretty heavily on your behavior and your health."

Noting that there is controversy over whether physicians should have access to this kind of data, Van Goor says that this information can work in the patient's favor. "It can be vital in helping your physician understand you better, and provide better treatment," he explains. "Are you a couch potato or are you somebody who goes to the gym regularly? The magazines that you read—whether you subscribe to *Runners Daily* or Barbecue *Daily*—say a lot about you. Where you go out to eat—all this stuff reflects on who you are as a person and what motivates you. I think potentially that has a huge effect on your health and your doctor should know that."

Admittedly, we would have to monitor a lot of seemingly disparate data points in order to pinpoint those that would be meaningful in terms of predicting health behaviors and outcomes. Every Big Data company contends that it alone has the secret sauce to home in on the right data and, using their proprietary analytic models, identify problem patients before they spiral out of control. Investors like Khosla Ventures, Kleiner Perkins, Flybridge Capital Partners and Flare Capital Partners are keen on these companies because this is very valuable information for payers, ACOs, providers and anyone who wants to intervene early in a patient's care in order to prevent a costly treatment, hospitalization or a fine by Medicare for rehospitalization.

There's no question that the practice of mining people's data to assess health risks is fraught with controversy. Privacy advocates are wary of the potential for abuse of personal health information by both payers and employers. There is also a raging debate over who owns your data, and how much say an individual should have in terms of how that information is used. Furthermore, there is a growing concern that hackers and others with ill intent could access private information. Major hospitals and insurers are not immune to security breaches, and all of this has left the public a bit uneasy.

One of the problems is that we've done a bad job educating society. It's pretty clear why all stakeholders would eagerly embrace predictive analytics as a new tool to improve outcomes and prevent expensive and avoidable episodes. The argument that hasn't been made—at least persuasively—is how individuals can benefit from the smart use of this data. Predictive analytics is not just about improving the bottom line for payers and providers, but enhancing quality of life by averting major health problems, promoting wellness and better engaging consumers in their own health based on individual lifestyle and personal preferences. This could be a win/win for providers, insurers and consumers, as long as it's done with transparency and integrity. (I cover this topic in depth in Chapter 12, The Privacy Trade-Offs.)

MAKING SENSE OF ALL THAT DATA

Despite the progress being made in using data to better understand human behavior and predict health outcomes, there are limitations to what it can do. For one thing, we are a society in data overload. There is so much data now available on each one of us, it's hard to discern what's meaningful and what isn't. *There are huge opportunities for businesses in this area. One is getting us from the sentence "People like Joe did [blank]" to "I know Joe so well, I can predict with certainty he'll behave in a certain way depending on the stimulus."*

And then, there's the next, important step—*making data actionable.* There are huge opportunities here as well. Identifying a problem is one thing; figuring out the personalized solution for each individual is another. The apt analogy here is, "You can lead a horse to water but you can't make him drink." If I can use our data-rich environment to formulate a package of attributes unique to you and a series of behaviors that have high probability of improving your health, but I can't engage you with a compelling message, it's all for naught.

Predictive analytics is not a crystal ball; not even the best-built algorithm can predict with a high degree of certainty the diagnosis of cancer or the sudden onset of an illness for which the patient had no risk factors, symptoms or unusual lab results. One day, a more sophisticated understanding of personal genomics may help explain some of these medical mysteries. Once we can combine the data streams of all of a person's phenotypic data (as we've been discussing) with the context of that person's genomic data, we will have a powerful data set on which to make even finer predictions.

Right now, predictive analytics can, with a reasonable degree of accuracy, identify changes in behavior—some fairly subtle—that could anticipate the worsening of a chronic or preexisting illness down the road. Some of this is pretty basic. For example, if an 80-year-old woman who has voted in every major election since she turned 21 doesn't show up at the polls, it could be a sign that she is having difficulty getting around, has become disconnected from the community or is having cognitive issues.

Even the actions of family members can point to a potential health crisis. Chris Coloian, senior vice president of CaféWell Insights, a division of Welltok, Inc., and the founder and president of Predilytics, a Burlington, Massachusetts, company that was recently acquired by Welltok, notes that a sudden uptick in how often family members contact their health plan about caregiver support and the available benefits is often a good indicator of impending acute risk. And according to Coloian, simply monitoring this interaction between a patient's family and their payer can result in a 15% to 20% improvement in predicting future hospitalizations.

As described on the company's website, "Predilytics applies patented, machine-learning analytic tools to transform our clients' structured and unstructured data, along with external data sources, into actionable insights." In addition to using healthcare payer and provider data, Predilytics, like other big data companies, uses publicly available data that include consumer, demographic, financial and clinical sources to create a fuller picture of the patient as a human being.

As Coloian describes it, predictive analytics has the potential to be the ultimate form of preventive medicine, enabling providers to intervene before a health problem takes hold. "We always knew that the best predictor of future cost was current cost utilization—actuaries have known that for years," he explains. "We also knew that people with chronic illnesses have a clinical cascade, which means that they were getting more care, year after year, as their health deteriorated. But it also turns out that there are early warning signs when we could intervene and hospitalization may be avoided, depending on underlying socioeconomic issues." According to Coloian, the difference today is that computer science is enabling healthcare to look beyond "a single pointed outcome and also view components of that outcome and ask, 'Where are the twists in the road, where are things going to change?'"

He explains further, "We've always been good at looking at mathematical relationships to high-volume events. What we haven't been really good at is breaking those down into component predictions and then looking at ways to modify the outcome. So not only do we want to identify somebody who is at risk for hospitalization, but we also want to know, is it an ambulatory-sensitive issue that's driving it? If you provided a program or resource to this person, which program or resource would mitigate it? If you provided the program or resource, would they engage with it?"

Presumably, once a payer or provider is alerted to a potential problem, it can take steps to offer assistance to the family or review the patient's current treatment. And that is precisely what payers and providers are banking on. Not just being able to predict when a chronic health problem could result in an expensive hospitalization, but finding effective ways to intervene and better engage patients to avert the potential crisis.

In this regard, healthcare can borrow a page or two from the playbook used by financial service companies that have long understood, when it comes to "engagement," one size doesn't fit all. Dr. Nick van Goor, who has a background in banking, says that financial services operate under the assumption that you need an understanding of what motivates an individual and then you tailor your approach accordingly. For example, when a consumer misses a credit card payment, a bank will consider several factors about the person before deciding the best approach, or "treatment," as it is called.

As Van Goor explains it, a lot of analytics are at work behind the scenes to decide what the bank should do about a missed payment, because individuals react differently to different stimuli. "For some people, it's best to leave them alone—it's called 'self cure.' The next month, when they realize they missed a payment, they'll pay double," he says. But he adds, "There's another group that are so far behind in their payments, there's no use throwing good money after bad, so banking institutions don't do anything about them. Then, there's a group in the middle; you want to understand them in order to figure out which 'treatments' you want to apply. Should you call them or send them a text? Or do you leave them alone for 10 days and then give them a call, or do you send them an email? There's a whole bunch of things you can do and different individuals react differently to the type of stimulus you do apply."

Providers are often faced with the same dilemma, except we don't get to dismiss the difficult cases as too hard to treat. We are obligated to care for everyone. That's why it's even more critical that we find ways to engage people early in the process and create tools to connect with each patient on a personal level. Practitioners have had to rely on intuition in order to determine the best approach for each patient, but it's difficult to learn about someone in a brief 10 to 20 minute yearly encounter.

Having a broader knowledge of a person's behavior patterns could be invaluable in terms of guiding a physician, says Partners' senior director Susan Lane. She recalls reading about a study conducted a few years ago that found that people who didn't wear their seat belts were more likely to be risk-takers. "It was very controversial because there was a suggestion that they should pay higher healthcare premiums," she says.

Although seat belt use isn't directly related to health, Lane thought that this information could be useful to providers in terms of better understanding an individual's mindset. "For example, we could predict that people who are risk-takers are more likely to be no-shows for their medical appointments. With that knowledge, when that patient is in the office, you would try to get as much done as possible and assume that they may not be coming back for a follow-up visit. And you may have to go into more detail about what they need to do on their own," she explains.

Bill Geary, whose company Flare Capital Partners was an investor in Predilytics and Explorys (now part of IBM), and who invested in Humedica (now part of Optum) with his former company, North Bridge Venture Partners, also believes healthcare analytics combined with connected health will enable physicians to better tailor their interactions with individual patients. "How do you motivate the sedentary diabetic to get off the couch? No one has yet cracked the code on how to change behavior for consumers or physicians when it comes to healthcare. Certain things will work for some of the people some of the time, and other things will work for other people at other times—the point being healthcare behavior change is intensely personal and requires unusual customization flexibility," he says. "What the industry needs is a full suite of not just the data, but also the predictive analytics that form actionable insights at the patient level. This allows providers to understand how people behaved previously, and why they did so, to help inform how they're going to behave in the future. The more you can personalize it, the more you can customize it for the individual, the more accurate it will be and the better it will be at altering behavior."

Chris Coloian believes that understanding personal preferences, to the point of knowing what time a person prefers to be contacted by a provider, can be the difference between a successful interaction and one that is viewed as intrusive. Says Coloian, "If you know someone prefers not to be called on weekends or after 7:00 at night, if an individual responds more quickly to a text versus email, then you're going to use those communication tools appropriately, right? You're going to use them in a way that is mindful and respectful to that consumer's needs."

The bottom line, Coloian says, is that consumers leave a good trail to what their probability or likelihood to engage is, as well as to what they will respond to. The problem is, healthcare hasn't been looking for these clues, until now. "This homogeneous, one-size-fits-all approach is not the way the world really works," he notes. "Actually, as populations go, we're very heterogeneous. It's not that engagement is tricky, it's when you have only one way to engage that engagement becomes tricky."

So how do we make sense of this opportunity? I think of it in three buckets of innovation:

Data gathering. This is the opportunity to collect all of the digital bread crumbs we have been talking about throughout this chapter, aggregate them and most importantly normalize them. The latter is a real innovation opportunity. We once hatched an exciting plan with a pharmacy chain, a consumer goods company, a pharmaceutical company and a firm expert in analytics to develop personas of people who had gone through the pharmacy. Were there relationships, for instance, between sports drink purchases and certain pharmaceutical purchases? Great vision, but after several months of discovery work we abandoned the project. We realized that one of the challenges would be that we just couldn't normalize all of those data sets. While I can aggregate my Withings weight scale data and my Fitbit activity data on the same app, they don't make internal sense when compared, because there is no mechanism to normalize them.

Analytics. As I've said, there are lots of companies working on this, but they haven't gotten close to predicting at the individual level. This is critical for success if we're going to really leverage analytics in healthcare.

Engagement. For me, this one is the most interesting areas. We have a vague sense of how advertisers are targeting ads in a very refined way based on our history of online behavior. This new world of advertising has made Facebook and Google (to name a couple) into corporate giants because those targeted ads generate a high number of spontaneous purchases compared to the old world of print ads and billboards. However, we know that getting you to take up and sustain a health-improving behavior is much more challenging than getting you to make an impulse purchase. There is an opportunity here to combine the lessons learned from the worlds of motivational psychology (Transtheoretical, Patient Activation Measure, Mindfulness, and so on), behavioral economics (choice architecture, nudges, and so on) and advertising/marketing (as far as I can tell the experts in all of these fields never compare notes) to create individualized, engaging messaging that will lead to sustained behavior change and improved health.

• • •

IF MOBILE PHONES COULD TALK

A mobile phone can tell a great deal about its user—whom she calls and who calls her; how long she chats with people; where she's traveled (thanks to GPS); her app usage; and how often she sends or receives texts or emails or interacts on other social media. Ginger.io, a startup San Francisco company, uses smartphone activity and predictive models developed by MIT scientists and engineers to assess an individual's mental health state and deliver more personalized care.

According to Karan Singh, co-founder of Ginger.io, whom I quote at the start of this chapter, we all have a daily pattern showing how we use our phones. A variation in a pattern could indicate a change in mental health status. "For example," says Singh, "in the case of depression, our models can detect a change in social isolation. The system might detect whether someone was communicating with fewer people, screening more calls, or wasn't interacting with their social network as much. *The key for us is to not only collect lots of data, but to actually map that to clinically relevant indicators of mental health conditions.*"

Some 40 medical centers, including Kaiser Permanente and the University of California, San Francisco, are offering the Ginger.io app for patients to track changes in behavior that could suggest worsening of a mental health problem, like depression, anxiety, a bipolar disorder or schizophrenia. "Our customers are looking to achieve better patient satisfaction, better clinical quality and lower cost," Singh explains.

For now, Singh says, Ginger.io's core use is for anxiety and depression. "Many people do not have enough access to the healthcare system to get the help they need. To make matters worse, there is currently no objective, physiological data available—there's no blood test for depression," he says. "The medical industry is built around paper-based self-reported surveys, and that's the gold standard for assessing mental health states. Much of what we're doing is digitizing that process and converting data we collect passively over a mobile device in order to identify when a patient may be slipping into a poor mental health state and then delivering the right intervention or proven coping strategy at the right time."

The Ginger.io app, available for iOS and Android, may be offered by providers, or individuals can download the app on their own. Users are first given a standard nine-question self-assessment survey through the app to evaluate levels of depression and anxiety. Once the baseline is established and users have downloaded the app, it begins to collect data about user behavior. According to Singh, "There are a series of interventions and support management programs we provide that are personalized based on the data we collect on an individual patient."

Singh notes that the movement away from fee-for-service to new payment models and population health has been a boon for Ginger.io. In particular, Singh says Ginger.io has been adopted by care management teams who are trying to be more proactive with their patients. "They can no longer just rely on self-reported data that comes in once or twice a year; they're doing location outreach to patients and looking at a series of different data," he explains. "We not only provide insights to those patients, but we can provide insights to therapists who can be reviewing their data along with their EMRs as part of their clinical consult."

Singh adds that the Affordable Care Act expands the Mental Health Parity and Addiction Equity Act (MHPAEA) of 2008, requiring health insurers and group health plans to provide the same level of benefits for mental and/or substance use treatment as for medical/surgical care. The problem is, there is a shortage of psychiatrists and other mental health professionals. According to the Health and Human Resources Administration, as of September 2014, about 96.5 million Americans were living in areas with shortages of mental health providers.

As a result, there's a growing interest among providers to leverage technologies like Ginger.io to meet the needs of this expanding group of patients. "By offering these coping tools, which allow patients to self-manage their condition, and by helping providers understand which of their patients need the most support, we can be that additional resource that can deliver better insight as to where providers should allocate their limited resources and spend their time," Singh says.

Ginger.io users range in age from 18-year-olds suffering from clinical depression or anxiety to 80-year-olds struggling with depression related to diabetes. If you're wondering if Ginger.io is an effective tool for older people who may not be as attached to their mobile phones as younger patients, you wouldn't be alone. Even the company founders were initially surprised to find that, while older people may use their phones less, they still have a pattern and when they deviate from that pattern, it could be a sign of a problem.

Citing the strong link between mental health and physical health, Singh notes that Ginger.io is participating in the Health eHeart Study being conducted at the University of California, San Francisco, to explore the role of behavioral data in predicting heart disease in those who don't yet have it. The Health eHeart Study is aiming to enroll one million patients. Study end points will include some physiological data, like EEG readings taken by a smartphone, as well as passive behavior data collected via Ginger.io.

According to Singh, "There is a huge co-morbidity associated with the top four physical health conditions—diabetes, heart failure, COPD and asthma—and mental health. It could be that up to 40% to 70% of patients with one of these chronic diseases also have a mental health issue that contributes meaningfully to patient outcomes. Some studies have shown that the actual cost of treating a patient with a chronic health condition, who also has a mental health issue, is double. If you support mental health, you also improve their physical health."

10

The Reinvention of Big Pharma

"Within the next decade, most prescribed drugs—especially for serious, chronic conditions—are going to come with a digital component, which we call connected therapies. It could be as basic as an app that connects you to a health coach who will guide you through how to take your medications and then help you stay adherent. Or, it could be as complex as a smart wearable sensor that monitors how you're doing and how you react to the drugs that you're taking. But it won't be the way it is today, with consumers being told, 'Oh, by the way, you can download an app with this drug if you want to.' The digital piece will be an important component of the prescription."

—RICK VALENCIA, SENIOR VICE PRESIDENT AND GENERAL MANAGER, QUALCOMM LIFE

The Big Shakeup has shaken up Big Pharma to its very core. On the surface, the prognosis isn't good.

I have spent countless hours behind closed doors listening to pharmaceutical executives bemoan the loss of their patents and express anxiety over the lack of potential blockbusters in the drug pipeline and new reimbursement models that favor generics over the pricier (and more profitable) name brands.

As I sit in these meetings, however, I can't help but feel that many of these pharma executives are missing the forest for the trees. It is easy to excuse this behavior. The pharmaceutical industry has been the beneficiary of high profit margins for many years. Yes, there is much risk in the early phases of the process—from discovery to a marketable product—but once a marketable product exists, patent law has allowed these companies to set prices and achieve monopoly status for their products, in some cases for decades. Companies typically recruit executives who have been successful in existing business models, so you can see why these folks are culturally and intellectually hamstrung with their current plight.

A big part of their market success has involved building relationships with others in their supply chain, most importantly prescribers. When I started my career, it was quite common for a nurse or receptionist to come into the clinic area where I'd be working and say that the rep from XYZ Company was in the waiting room and would I be willing to spend five minutes with him/her? I usually obliged. During my five minutes, I got the carefully rehearsed pitch about their latest products and some branded leave-behinds like coffee mugs or sticky pads. Once that relationship was established, the rep would often stop by with sports tickets or dinner invitations. I never took part in these more obvious bribes, but I prescribed my share of new products as a result of these in-office interactions.

In large part, what made this method of product sales successful for the pharma industry is that we never discussed price. Generics were not a big deal and it was pretty easy for these sales reps to come up with cogent reasons for why we should prescribe branded products anyway. Insurers and their plan sponsors (employers) were left out in the cold as the pharma industry cozied up to prescribers and together drove up the cost of care.

Fast forward to 2015—it has been several years since I've met with a pharmaceutical rep. In the meantime, as our organization has become more value-conscious (value is outcomes divided by costs), we've looked carefully at our suppliers to see how we could squeeze costs out of the supply chain. Pharmaceuticals were an early easy target.

Beginning about seven years ago, and continuing today, whenever I write a prescription in my EMR, I am chastised if I write it for a branded product. I get many cheerful reminders about the cost of branded products vs. generics. As a consequence, I almost never prescribe branded products anymore (except in the area of specialty pharma and I'll shortly get to that). Oh, how the world has changed! Add to this the fact that consumers are now paying higher copays and higher deductibles and getting constant feedback themselves on costs, and how all of the pharmacy chains (starting with Walmart in 2006) now offer generic drugs for a few dollars per 90-day supply, and you can see how the world of Big Pharma is collapsing.

When panicked, most human beings tend to focus on routine behaviors that are almost instinctive. So, here we are back at the problem of not seeing the forest for the trees. Pharma executives need to take a broader view and, as the saying goes, try to make lemonade out of lemons.

This chapter will focus on the market trends that are changing the dynamics of this industry; how in the era of mobile and ubiquitous connectivity, software tools can have an impact as good as or better than some medications; and how certain companies are already on the journey to creating this bold new future.

TWO TRENDS TO WATCH

Let's start out with the two seemingly opposing trends in healthcare that are having a profound impact on the future of the pharmaceutical industry:

First, the move to value-based, outcomes-based payment models and population health management is shining a spotlight on the critical need to reduce spending and improve medication adherence. As noted above, when providers take on risk for population health, they start to scrutinize their costs of providing care. One easy, painless target for them is to better control pharmaceutical costs.

And, almost as a countervailing force, there has been explosive growth in "specialty pharmaceuticals," the crop of molecules called "biologics" that are developed via biotechnology. These drugs are complex to manufacture, require special handling and care coordination, and are astronomically expensive. You can think of the process of prescribing these drugs as an investment on some-body's part (whoever is the risk-bearer). In the same way you look after your mutual funds and your 401(k), the people making an investment in these ex-pensive drugs want to make sure they are being used in a way that maximizes the investment. This creates a great interest in adherence.

So, in very different ways, both of these trends present huge opportunities for potentially *profitable* connected health solutions.

Like everything else in healthcare these days, it comes down to proving your worth. This call to action will probably be magnified in the case of Big Pharma, but these questions apply to all participants in the value chain: Are you keeping patients healthy and out of the hospital? Are you preventing high-risk patients from spiraling out of control? Are you helping ACOs, population health groups and other healthcare organizations cut costs and still provide quality care? Most importantly, if you are not, you are likely to be marginal-ized or commoditized.

Big Pharma may think that it can operate under different rules—and for years it did. But those days are long gone.

Greg Barrett, vice president of Marketing and Managed Markets at Daiichi Sankyo (DSI), summed it up beautifully at the 2015 ePharma Summit in New York City. "If a pharma company today is not thinking about how to inte-grate, not just use as a tool to promote, but integrate programs and education resources around the pill and the bottle, you will be left behind," Barrett said. "We are all going to be measured by our ability to increase value, to increase the quality of care and lower costs."

That's a tall order considering that the most exciting pharmaceutical breakthroughs are coming from the biotech sector and are hitting our pock-etbooks hard. By 2017, close to *half* the amount of money we spend on drugs in the United States will be on so called "specialty pharmaceuticals." Biologics have revolutionized how we can treat conditions like hepatitis C, rheumatoid arthritis (RA), multiple sclerosis, psoriasis and many different types of cancer. They offer new hope to millions of people suffering from these and other conditions, and the demand for biologics is expected to keep growing.

This progress has come with a steep price tag. Gilead Sciences' blockbuster drug Solvadi, a breakthrough cure for hepatitis C, costs $84,000 for a 12-week treatment or a whopping $1,000 a pill. The annual cost for Amgen's Enbrel, used by rheumatoid arthritis (RA) and psoriasis patients, can reach upwards of $39,000. And the average cost of oncology agents has doubled over the past decade from $5,000 to $10,000 a month. Although the U.S. Food and Drug Administration (FDA) recently approved the sale of the first generic biologic (called a biosimilar) to treat RA, most of these therapies are patent protected, which means the price won't be going down for years.

Drug prices across the board are rising so fast that physicians are beginning to rebel against prescribing some of the pricier therapeutics. In May 2014, Bloomberg.com ran the ominous headline (for Big Pharma, that is), "Cancer Doctors Join Insurers in U.S. Drug-Cost Revolt," with an article that described how physicians at Memorial Sloan Kettering Cancer Center in New York City publicly criticized the skyrocketing prices for new chemotherapy drugs. In July 2015, 118 oncologists from throughout the United States signed an editorial, published in *Mayo Clinic Proceedings*, protesting the high cost of chemotherapy drugs.

According to a survey by Bloomberg, "Dozens of medicines for ailments ranging from cancer to multiple sclerosis, diabetes and high cholesterol have doubled or more in price since late 2007." The Bloomberg review used data supplied by DRX, a Milwaukee, Wisconsin–based company that provides drug comparison information. Not exactly great publicity for the industry.

AN RX FOR BEHAVIOR CHANGE

At the same time that we've made enormous strides in the treatment of some very difficult conditions, we still have persistent lifestyle issues—such as inactivity, overeating, smoking and the like—which can stifle this progress and that can't be solved in a laboratory.

It's no secret that medication adherence is a huge problem—some studies suggest about 50% of patients don't take their medications as directed. This can get very costly. A 2013 report by CVS Caremark estimated that poor medication adherence costs the U.S. healthcare system up to $290 billion annually in additional treatment, including visits to the ER and hospital stays. This is money that could have been saved if only people took their medications as prescribed.

There are numerous reasons why people don't take their medications, but often it comes down to not really understanding why they need them in the first place. As I've noted earlier, many of the most insidious chronic conditions, like high blood pressure and prediabetes, are symptomless until they have caused a good deal of damage in the body. Patients simply don't believe that they're sick enough to need drugs when they're feeling fine. The 10-minute discussion they had in the doctor's office about their condition may have been quickly forgotten by the time they got home. Additionally, even well-meaning patients who strive to follow instructions may simply not understand them. For example, when a newly discharged patient winds up back in the ER or rehospitalized as a result of not taking his meds properly, it is often due to the fact that he (or his caregiver) didn't fully comprehend the treatment protocol when he left the hospital. Or it could be that the prescription is very complicated, contains multiple pills and requires special care. At times, patients may be fearful of the meds side effects if they are not well explained.

Whether it's a $2 generic or a blockbuster biologic molecule with a five (or six) figure price tag, it's important for people to take their medications properly for their own safety and well-being. From the perspective of the payer, however, it is particularly imperative that a patient follow his or her prescription regimen when taking an expensive biologic. Poor adherence to these pricey drugs can result in tens of thousands of dollars literally being washed down the drain.

For example, among our hepatitis C patient population, self-reported adherence to Solvadi is 85%, which I might add is great considering that a 50% compliance rate is much more the norm. It does suggest, however, that 15% of the time, these individuals are not following the prescribed treatment protocol. The problem with a therapy like Solvadi is if a patient misses his pills for three days in a row, he has to start the entire regimen all over again. And at $1,000 a pill, that can become very costly, very quickly. Once again, the analogy of investment is applicable—the individual making this investment will want to see a return.

The bottom line: *These two trends—the move to drive down healthcare costs and the rise of expensive specialty pharmaceuticals—have created an urgent need for better patient engagement and improved medication adherence. What better way to achieve this than with a digital component that is with the consumer 24/7 and that can provide immediate information and support to improve outcomes and reduce costs.*

It is now a cliché to say, "Big Pharma needs to start thinking 'beyond the pill,'" but this is exactly the challenge. It's true that every drug developer may not strike gold with a billion dollar blockbuster. But with its access to patients and marketing expertise, Big Pharma could be selling something that is even more valuable to payers and providers—consumer engagement.

There is a new, untapped, potentially profitable business model for pharma: The molecule becomes the loss leader and surrounding services that lead to better compliance and healthier patients become the revenue source. Larry Brooks, director of Business Development, Digital Health, and his team at Boehringer Ingelheim, were some of the first in the industry to start thinking beyond the pill. In fact, several of our pharma clients are preparing to release new drugs that come with a prescription for a lifestyle/compliance program for patients. Later in this chapter, I'll describe a joint project that we are working on with one of them.

For the most part, however, Big Pharma has ceded this territory to non-pharma companies like Samsung, which have moved in quickly to secure this lucrative market. Samsung, primarily known as a leading tech company, is making a heavy investment in generic drug companies producing biosimilar drugs, which are biologic drugs that have lost their patent. Analysts are already predicting that Samsung will soon dominate the generic market. How? By adding health and wellness programs that lead to better compliance and presumably strong consumer loyalty.

Walgreens is an example of a company currently making $325 million dollars a month just on its mobile health support services alone. Every dollar Walgreens makes on selling prescription support services is lost revenue for

Big Pharma. Another example is CVS. In addition to running its retail/pharmacy and MinuteClinics, CVS Health, a health benefits plan manager for 60 million Americans, is launching a Digital Innovation Lab in Boston.

A *BETTER* PILL TO SWALLOW

Proteus Digital Health, a Redwood City, California–based company founded in 2001, is an example of a sizzling hot "New Pharma" company that doesn't produce, discover or develop a single drug in the conventional sense. Last February, the company was featured as part of the *Wall Street Journal's* Billion Dollar Startup Club, a select group of private companies valued at over $1 billion by venture capitalists. What Proteus is selling is adherence, engagement and effectiveness.

The Proteus "service offering," as the company calls it, is comprised of an ingestible sensor and a tiny silicon chip that is integrated with a medicine. A separate patch, worn like a Band-Aid on the patient's torso, tracks activity, rest, and heart rate, and also when the integrated Digital Medicine is taken. The patch relays the data to the patient's mobile device and the information can also be accessed by the patient's care team in a secure web-based portal. Data analytics–based services are provided by Proteus to patients and healthcare teams to personalize pharmaceutical therapy and make it more effective in treating patients to therapeutic goals.

The Proteus sensor contains two common minerals normally found in food and the human body—magnesium and copper—which interact with stomach acid to produce a heartbeat-like signal that is detected by the patch. In other words, the system is self-powered by the body. Hence the Proteus slogan, "We believe in health care, powered by you." In 2012, the FDA cleared the Proteus ingestible sensor as a medical device; it has also been cleared for use in Europe. The Proteus service offering is being evaluated and used commercially in the United States and by the National Health Service (NHS) in the United Kingdom.

The Proteus system is far more than an ingestible tracker that polices drug adherence, however. The beauty of the Proteus patch is that it monitors other biometrics that may be of clinical relevance, including activity level, steps walked, body position, temperature, sleep patterns and heart rate variability. This information, along with medication adherence data, can support patient self-care and physician decision making.

Interestingly, Proteus's ability to integrate medication-taking patterns with daily lifestyle decisions is the aspect of the system that has resonated with Paul L., a 52-year-old patient living in London who is participating in a pilot program through the NHS.

After Paul suffered a heart attack and had open-heart surgery, his doctor warned him that he would have to become more vigilant about his health or risk having another heart attack. He was advised to get more exercise, lose weight and carefully adhere to his medication schedule, which meant taking multiple medications carefully spaced throughout the day. In addition to managing his own condition, Paul is also the primary caregiver for his wife, who is confined to a wheel chair due to severe arthritis. Paul remembers leaving the hospital feeling very scared, depressed and overwhelmed.

Despite his uncertainty for a successful recovery, four months after his surgery, when we spoke with Paul by phone, he was not only back at work, but 10 pounds lighter and feeling fitter than he had in decades. Since his surgery, he had not only lost weight but had become much more conscious about adding activity to his day. Paul attributes his ability to bounce back quickly to the Proteus service offering, which he says has steered him to a healthier lifestyle. "It (Proteus) can see if I'm sitting too much, it can see if I'm moving around, and it can see how well I'm sleeping," Paul explains. "My goal is to walk at least 10,000 steps a day, but I try to do better. I check my numbers throughout the day and if I see that I'm falling short, I make it up."

The word that Paul uses the most to describe the Proteus program is "motivation." Without it, he says he wouldn't have been driven to take an extra walk at night, bypass the "lift" to climb up the five flights of stairs to his apartment in order to log extra steps or seek out places to walk indoors when the weather is damp and cold.

Now that Paul is back at work, he needs to take his medication with him for his midday dose, which he admits could easily be forgotten if he is otherwise distracted. He counts on the patch to keep track for him. "It reminds me if I forget to take my tablets," he says. "It's made my life a lot less stressful. There's no question that it has changed my life for the better."

Paul is representative of tens of millions of people in the United States and throughout the world who are coping with multiple medical problems that require good medication adherence as well as significant lifestyle changes. These are often the patients who are at high risk of not taking their medications as prescribed. These are also the patients who are most likely to wind up being rehospitalized or who end up in the ER in crisis.

In a world where compliance is such a pressing issue, a tool like the Proteus offering could be useful in helping physicians and nurses understand whether patients are progressing toward their therapy goal or are in need of an intervention. Proteus's chief product officer, David O'Reilly, offers an even bigger vision for Proteus—as a tool for "self-knowledge and self-actuation" and ultimately behavior change.

O'Reilly explains that, "With these data-driven insights, people can begin to connect behavior choices—some really important ones—around medication-taking behavior, body movement decisions and patterns, and sleep quality decisions and patterns. For example, we might help someone notice that when he gets a certain number of hours of sleep per night, he is more likely to take his medication than when he doesn't get enough sleep. Or that, for some reason, Tuesdays are the worst days for him to try to keep on track with his medicines or other lifestyle choices."

O'Reilly also points out that the ability to form these kinds of insights goes well beyond the usual data feeds and alerts that people often quickly tune out. "The goal here is to get to habit formation, which is more often linked to different types of intrinsic and extrinsic rewards and incentives than to just alerts with nothing else," he says.

Proteus is not just looking at how a drug works in the body, but how humans interact with and react to the drug so patients can make the kind of nonpharmaceutical changes in their behavior that will enhance their health. Simply put, it's not about the pill—a new reality that O'Reilly feels the pharma industry has not yet grasped. "The pharmaceutical industry still thinks it has to base everything in digital health around the stature of the brand, the individual molecule," he says. "That's not what health systems want to buy, or patients care about. What patients care about is, 'How do I treat this condition when I'm on five to 15 medicines and I have one to four different comorbid conditions?' We believe that is how one needs to think about digital medicines and a digital health offering around them. Because it's not about the drug, and it's not about the disease, it's about the consumer, their situation and their collaboration with physicians and nurses."

Proteus could very well be the model for the pharmaceutical company of the future. By that I'm not suggesting that it will turn its attention to creating the next billion-dollar molecule. Rather, it could offer behavior and lifestyle modification programs, partnered with a suite of generic drugs, that will connect with consumers in a way that has not been done before.

In this model, the drug really does become the loss leader and the ability to engage consumers becomes the profit center.

At Partners Connected Health, we've had quite a few of our own "beyond the pill" success stories. One of the most interesting is a clinical research program we recently completed with adolescents who have asthma, a very tough patient population. Teenage asthmatics are notoriously difficult patients who feel invincible (just like others their age), ignore symptoms and don't take their medications as directed. As a result, the typical asthmatic teen will land in the emergency department three times a year at a cost of $6,000 per incident, not to mention the emotional wear and tear on their families.

To help improve compliance, we created a private Facebook group for these teens. No fancy bells and whistles—just old-fashioned social networking. The study is now closed and we are still reviewing the data, but to date we've already seen a positive effect, as measured by an instrument called the Asthma Control Test (ACT). Typically, the success rate of teenagers filling out this survey is 18%. Although the results are still preliminary, it appears that just putting kids in a Facebook group increased their participation to 80%. More importantly, according to the ACT measures, how well these teens are controlling their asthma also appears to be significantly improved, compared with the use of a new inhaler.

To me, what was even more impressive was the fact that when the study was completed, the participants begged us to extend it. We went back to the Institutional Review Board (IRB) on their behalf and were able to keep it going a bit longer than planned. So it seems that Facebook can be more therapeutic than a drug! Social networking could be the key to significantly improving medication adherence for certain segments of the population, and it doesn't require any expensive technology.

We're also testing an app that is designed to help cancer patients better manage their pain. It's a small study but an important one. Some 80% to 90% of cancer patients suffer from pain, but the problem is often underreported and undertreated, for several reasons. Some patients are embarrassed to admit that they are in pain; others believe that pain is an essential part of their recovery. But this is not just a quality of life issue—a substantial number of patients stop chemotherapy due to pain, which can be life threatening. Although palliative medication is available, patients may run out and forget to reorder it until they suddenly need it, and then have to go through the process of calling their doctor and having the prescription renewed, all of which takes time.

Our cancer pain management app enables patients to easily report their pain, find tools to better cope it, and reorder their pain medication. First, patients are asked to rate their pain levels three times a week on the app's pain scale. In addition to being given tips on how to better manage their pain, patients are also reminded to reorder their medication and can do so by simply tapping the screen to notify their provider. So far, we have found that the self-reporting of pain among app users is 80%, considerably higher than the 30% to 35% typical among cancer patients. We've also seen an improvement in overall pain scores, as improved pain reporting is associated with better pain relief. And, patients who better manage pain control use fewer resources.

A NEW WAY TO LAUNCH A DRUG

In collaboration with Partners Connected Health, Daiichi Sankyo has stepped up to the plate to change the way pharmaceuticals are impacting the marketplace. We have jointly developed a mobile companion to usual drug therapy—an app for patients suffering from atrial fibrillation, the most common heart arrhythmia. Atrial fibrillation (AFib for short) is characterized by a glitch in the heart's electrical system that causes it to beat too fast or too slow, or with an irregular rhythm. This increases the risk for blood clots and stroke. Treatment for AFib involves using blood thinners to prevent the blood from becoming "sticky," or forming clots when it's not supposed to.

The launch of the app coincides with the FDA's approval of DSI's new drug Savaysa (edoxaban), a "novel oral anticoagulant," or NOAC. For decades, warfarin (marketed under the names Coumadin and Jantoven, for example), a vitamin K antagonist, was the only FDA-approved drug for the treatment of stroke prevention for AFib patients. In recent years, the FDA has approved three NOACs: Pradaxa (dabigatran), Xarelto (rivaroxaban) and Eliquis (apixaban). Savaysa makes four.

The DSI/Partners app can be used by any patient with AFib, regardless of what medication or treatment he is taking. It provides in-depth, impartial information on all available medications, without favoring one over another. The goal is to provide support to all patients living with atrial fibrillation by helping to improve patient adherence and compliance to medication, as well as fostering feedback loops that connect the provider to the patient.

The app allows patients to use their smartphone camera and light-emitting diode (LED), which can track heart rate as well as any episodes of arrhythmia as they are happening. This enables patients to see any connections between these episodes and their behaviors, like food intake, or with other medications they may be taking.

According to the FDA, some three million Americans have this condition, which typically occurs after age 65. As the population ages, so will the number of AFib cases. According to the American Heart Association, "Even though untreated atrial fibrillation doubles the risk of heart-related deaths and causes a four- to five-fold increased risk for stroke, many patients are unaware that AFib is a serious condition."

Like so many of the "stealth" diseases I've written about earlier, AFib is a prime example of an "out of sight, out of mind" ailment. Some people with AFib may have absolutely no symptoms; and even when people have symptoms, they may be fleeting. Typical symptoms include what is often described as a "fluttering" sensation in the chest, or patients may feel lightheaded or faint or have chest palpitations.

About 40% of people with AFib chose not to take any medication. During our research to develop the AFib app, we learned that many patients fail to understand the seriousness of the condition. They believe that they are only at risk for stroke when the heart is fibrillating, and this is not true. After even one episode, the risk for stroke remains higher than normal throughout their lifetime, whether or not they actually experience symptoms. We realized that there was a great deal of misinformation circulating about this condition and that there was a huge need for an impartial source of information.

The decision of which drug to take is a personal choice that needs to be made in the context of an individual's lifestyle. There are both risks and advantages for all AFib therapies that need to be understood. For example, people taking warfarin must have regular blood tests to make sure it is dosed correctly: If the dose is too low, it will be ineffective; if too high, it can cause excess bleeding. These patients also have to be extremely careful about their diet and avoid eating a lot of foods containing vitamin K, like leafy greens vegetables and legumes, which can interfere with the effectiveness of the therapy.

There are some advantages to NOACs over warfarin. Notably, there is a reduced risk of bleeding and, therefore, NOACs do not require frequent blood tests. Nor do patients have to worry about vitamin K consumption. So when these drugs were introduced, it was believed that they would require fewer lifestyle changes and that this would lead to superior compliance.

Recent studies may suggest that is not the case. Although NOACs are more convenient, eliminating regular blood tests may result in poor patient compliance. In other words, because nobody is watching, and the disease is basically silent, medication adherence may not be as good as originally expected. The problem is, despite the lack of symptoms, these patients are still at risk for stroke and really do need to be taking these medications consistently.

You may ask, what's in it for DSI to support an unbranded beyond the pill initiative? For one thing, ACOs and managed care organizations need new tools to promote medication adherence, but would not be receptive to an "information" app that was actually a marketing tool promoting one product. If DSI wanted their app to be widely used, it had to be generic.

Second, despite the fact that the app is generic, DSI sales reps will be promoting the app along with their new drug, which may indirectly help to brand their NOAC as consumer-friendly in the eyes of physicians.

Third, DSI is counting on the fact that once patients have the full story about AFib, many who are reluctant to take a medication may decide to try one. Of course, many patients may opt for other brands, but odds are, some may use DSI's offering. Furthermore, the better educated patients are about their condition, the more likely they are to use these medications properly and the less likely they are to run into trouble. An app like the one we designed can better help patients understand the need for compliance, as well as give providers a tool to monitor adherence.

One rule we have at Partners Connected Health is that we only work with companies and on projects where we can see downstream value for our delivery system. In this case, we were intrigued by the idea that using a more expensive therapeutic, combined with a more closely/tightly managed approach to the condition, might lead to better outcomes and lower overall costs. If this succeeds, it paves a path for specialty pharma in the context of the ACO.

THINKING OUTSIDE THE BOTTLE

For some real "beyond the pill, outside the bottle" thinking, look no further than the work being done by Durham, North Carolina–based BD Technologies, a leader in developing safe and easy-to-use injection devices. According to Noel G. Harvey, BD's vice president of Research and Development, the company, which sells in excess of 40 billion syringes and catheters annually, sees a big role for itself in digital medicine. "A few years ago, it became obvious to us that if we could make our very basic devices smart, so that they could collect data and then be analyzed, it could be a tremendous public health tool," Harvey explains.

At the time, Harvey was doing public policy work for BD in Washington, DC, around pandemic preparedness and there was concern over the spread of new types of flu. "There is great interest in how smart delivery systems and smart diagnostics could help with the containment of an epidemic like flu," he says. "If we could diagnose that someone had a certain strain of flu, we could then pinpoint where the outbreak was and verify that vaccinations had been given in the surrounding areas. By having the devices connected, we have a real public health tool that could have tremendous value."

To achieve this goal, BD is pioneering the development of "smart inject-ables" that can help patients and providers keep better track of medication adherence, as well as proper dosing. Harvey notes that BD has already proto-typed multiple platforms, but it's still very early in the process. According to Harvey, "For instance, we've made prototypes for insulin therapy for diabetics that could, in theory, calculate the correct dose for each individual at that precise time based on glucose readings. The device could then check to see if you want that dose. If you don't want that dose, it could ask what dose you do want. It then programs the right dose into the injector. All that information gets recorded in the device, in your cell phone or your tablet, and ostensibly it could be programmed into your EMR."

As Harvey observes, not only would this system titrate the right dose at that moment, but over time, this information could also help people to better understand chronic conditions like diabetes. "If you have diabetes, every day you prick your finger or you take your continuous glucose reading. Then you have to calculate your dose and give yourself your medication. That's basically the standard protocol right now. It's good therapy, but eventually complica-tions can arise. If a problem occurs, there's no record of what could be leading to those complications. With this system, you could collect the data, analyze the data so that you understand the pattern and then act on it," he says.

When you begin to think beyond the pill, as the people at BD are doing, the sky is the limit—and I mean this quite literally.

Using a drone that can be controlled by a tablet or smartphone, Harvey says his team at BD has actually prototyped a system for providing timely as-sistance to healthcare clinics in underserved areas like in sub-Saharan Africa and Haiti. Many areas like these not only suffer from a severe shortage of medical personnel, but the lack of refrigeration makes it difficult to store per-ishable medical supplies, like vaccines, or keep blood samples fresh.

In the BD prototype, an on-site health worker armed with a tablet and app could survey the population of a remote village to determine who needs what vaccine, medication or blood test and input this information onto the tablet.

As Harvey explains it, "The tablet or iPhone has an app that contains all the questions that the World Health Organization wants health workers to ask an individual patient during a vaccination clinic or care checkup." Once the information is collected, the data could be uploaded to the tablet, stored in the cloud and accessed from afar. From a different location, a drone could be loaded with precisely the supplies that are needed. The worker could control when the drone arrives so that the supplies could be used immediately, as opposed to sitting in the heat and going to waste. On the return trip, the drone could deliver the blood samples for analysis in a lab. This ingenious system would allow healthcare workers to travel from village to village and know that they would be able to get the resources they need with a swipe of a screen.

This may all still be in the development stage, but it is the type of innovation every pharmaceutical company should be thinking about.

There are really two ways for the pharmaceutical industry to move beyond the pill:

1. Bundle connected health solutions with molecules—the Daiichi example is a great one.
2. Radically rethink what it means to be in the business of providing therapeutics. We've shown that properly implemented software engagement tools can do as well as or better than a molecule at achieving health outcomes.

As good as the margins in pharma are, the margins for software can be even more attractive (Microsoft is worth more than any pharma company). That reinvention is possible, but it will require real leadership and a big upfront investment.

11

The Digital Rx

"Who would have thought, when we first embarked on pursuing a prescription for a mobile health product, that the winds of policy change would be blowing in our direction. WellDoc was never initially focused on reimbursement for a medical device, or a service—we were shifting the focus from a 'widget' to 'value.' Our belief was that mobile prescription therapy would be reimbursed for engagement, value and dare I say—outcomes!"

—ANAND IYER, PHD, MBA, CHIEF DATA SCIENCE OFFICER,
WELLDOC

Back in the twentieth century, we looked to medical miracles like antibiotic "wonder drugs" and vaccines to solve the most pressing health issues of the day. And, for the most part, they produced spectacular results. In 1900 America, the average life expectancy was 47 years old and one out of five children died before the age of five. A century later, we have increased the average life expectancy by more than three decades—a remarkable feat—and death in childhood is now a rare and tragic event. This evolution bred several generations of doctors who increasingly began to look at their patients from a physiologic, body-system perspective. It also bred a pharmaceutical industry that has made billions of dollars in profit-creating molecules that target organ pathology. Consumers, when they turned into patients, began to ask for a "pill" as the easy cure for any malady.

But, the reality is, although people are living longer, they are not necessarily living healthier. We are losing ground in terms of the so-called "health span." The net result of this focused physiologic approach on the part of all parties has been a loss of appreciation for both the person as a whole and for the importance of behavioral factors in caring for illness.

The rapid change in lifestyle that occurred during the twentieth century—the deadly combination of increased consumption of highly processed, high-calorie foods and a sedentary lifestyle—has produced a sharp rise in chronic illnesses. The word "epidemic," once used to describe contagious diseases like the flu and TB, is now regularly paired with conditions like "obesity" and "diabetes."

Here's the irony of it all: In our lifetime, it's unlikely that lifestyle-related diseases—like diabetes, obesity and heart disease—will be cured by taking a pill or giving yourself a shot. The reality is, the most effective treatments may be the more difficult ones to sustain, such as improving your diet, getting more sleep, increasing physical activity and maintaining a healthy weight. Enter the renaissance of behavioral interventions—we are relearning what our ancestors learned about the power of the mind to influence the course of illness.

The renewed emphasis on the power of the mind and the need to conquer chronic lifestyle-related illnesses create the opportunity for us to rethink what can go into an effective therapeutic. It's not just about molecules anymore; it's about digital therapeutics, or Digital Rx.

Even five years ago, the concept of investing in digital therapies to help prevent or better manage chronic conditions would have been considered well-meaning but naive. Today, the tables have turned. Payers and providers who believe that the economics haven't changed are the ones who have their heads in the clouds.

The new reality demands that providers and payers find ways to improve outcomes and efficiencies while cutting costs—goals that can only be achieved by boosting medication adherence and patient engagement. There is no one secret formula to achieving these goals. However, as discussed in Chapter 10, where I covered the changing pharmaceutical industry, the emerging trends involve the coupling of holistic packages of digital products with molecules—that is, programs that combine digital behavior change tools with medications in order to extend the reach of healthcare providers. Another trend to watch is programs that feature digital prescriptions alone—no drugs—like the Text2Move initiative for people with diabetes and the Facebook community for teen asthmatics, which I described earlier.

In this chapter, I take a closer look at three startup companies—Omada Health, WellDoc and Twine Health—that are developing digital tools to help people better manage chronic conditions, each with different perspectives and approaches. What they all have in common, however, is that they didn't take their products straight to consumers. These innovators didn't want to develop yet another weight loss app or online weight loss community. They wanted to leverage the power of digital to create a new category of treatment that would be scientifically based, medically approved and, most importantly, attractive to both providers and payers as a tool that could actually save money.

OMADA HEALTH: A DIGITAL THERAPEUTIC

Founded in 2011 by Sean Duffy and Adrian James, San Francisco–based Omada Health is a self-proclaimed "digital therapeutics" company. Duffy defines digital therapeutics as "taking the face-to-face behavior change programs that have been proven to be effective and bringing them to the digital era." Omada's flagship product, Prevent, is a digital curriculum based, in part, on the National Institute of Health's groundbreaking National Diabetes Prevention Program (NDPP).

In March 2015, for the first time in its history, the U.S. Centers for Disease Control officially recognized three digital programs—including Omada Health's Prevent—as meeting the evidence-based standards for the agency's National Diabetes Prevention Program.

Duffy and James cooked up the idea for the company while they were both working at IDEO, then a San Francisco–based design firm. Duffy was doing an internship as part of a joint MD/MBA program at Harvard; James led the Medical Products domain for IDEO's Health and Wellness Practice.

They targeted what they saw as a coming epidemic—obesity-related chronic conditions, largely driven by lifestyle, and largely preventable. As noted earlier, today chronic diseases kill more people worldwide than infectious diseases, and 75% of all Americans will die prematurely from diseases that could have been prevented through changes in lifestyle.

Take prediabetes. Today some 86 million American adults—37% of the US population—are prediabetic, a condition characterized by higher than normal blood sugar levels or, more specifically, HbA1c in the range of 5.7% to 6.4% (A1c of 6.5% or more is bona fide diabetes). Only one in 10 Americans with prediabetes is even aware that he or she has the condition. This isn't simply unfortunate, it's dangerous—prediabetes can lead not only to diabetes, but can also increase the risk of heart attack, stroke, kidney failure and even cancer. Prediabetes is very much a lifestyle-related disease, associated with obesity, lack of exercise and poor diet. The obvious cure is to lose weight, increase activity and eat better. Easy to say, but not so easy to do.

Prevent is a 16-week, online, interactive lifestyle intervention program that uses digital tools like a pedometer and a cellular-enabled scale to monitor progress. It also provides health coaches trained in the CDC's prevention program for weekly nutrition and fitness guidance, and offers an online support group of peers with whom you can share your data.

The program is available for participants via any laptop, tablet or smartphone. Participants are divided into groups of 12 individuals based on factors like location, weight loss goals, life stage and personality. Each group works with a health coach, who is available to answer questions via text, email or phone 24 hours a day, seven days a week. People who complete the four-month program graduate to a maintenance program called Sustain.

Not surprisingly, a company created by two IDEO alumni has made design a foundational element from the beginning. The interface is simple—the cellular-enabled scale and pedometer automatically sync to the user's private account—and the packaging is attractive. The median age of the Prevent user is 50 years old, and the fact that most users are not "digital natives" is always on Duffy's mind. From the get-go, the emphasis was on creating as seamless and streamlined a consumer experience as possible, which he feels has given Prevent a leg up over other digital weight loss programs. "I think of design as our small molecule—it's the thing that makes it work," Duffy says.

Duffy knows that losing weight and lowering blood sugar are not easy tasks, and people need to feel that they have an abundance of support helping them to make that happen. "It takes an extraordinary amount of effort to even get modest results, and that's just the reality. It's very hard to change your lifestyle," Duffy acknowledges. With that in mind, he says, "Our goal—and a requirement for our company—is to give every person the feeling that we're just dropping in the paratroopers to help them. They've got a clear goal, social support from their group, they can see how others are progressing in their group, there's a coach, they've got a scale that sends the data back, they've got a curriculum that engages them every step of the way—all wrapped in a design that they've never seen from a healthcare company."

Prevent uses all the tricks in the book to keep people engaged, including some unexpected rewards, like a motivational package with an attractive picture frame that shows up at the participant's door during the final weeks of the program. "We tell them to put a picture of a loved one in the frame to remind them why they're in the Prevent program," says Duffy.

All of this virtual handholding appears to be working as well or better than the conventional approach. Peer-reviewed, published studies have shown that Prevent can work as well or at times better at helping people maintain weight loss and control blood sugar as the face-to-face counseling administered under the NDPP program. One 2015 study, "Long-Term Outcomes of a Web-Based Diabetes Prevention Program: 2-Year Results of a Single-Arm Longitudinal Study," published in the *Journal of Medical Internet Research (JMIR)*, found that Prevent compared favorably to the NDPP in that, "Users of the *Prevent* program experienced significant reductions in body weight and A1c that are maintained after 2 years. Contrary to the expected progression from prediabetes to diabetes over time, average A1c levels continued to show an average regression from within the prediabetic range (5.7%-6.4%) initially to the normal range (<5.7%) after 2 years."

Prevent is primarily directed to employers, health plans and payers who offer the service to employees and beneficiaries. Pricing is based on the outcomes achieved by individuals. That is, Omada Health gets reimbursed based on how well people achieve and maintain their goals. Although Prevent doesn't spend any money marketing to individuals, the 16-week program is also offered to consumers for $120 per month.

The attractive, no-risk payment model is not the only reason why payers and providers are interested in funding a program that prevents diabetes. According to the American Diabetes Association, people diagnosed with diabetes incur average medical expenditures of about $13,700 per year, of which about $7,900 is attributed to diabetes. Every prediabetic patient who doesn't develop the disease represents real savings.

Omada Health was part of digital health accelerator Rock Health's inaugural class. Since its inception, the company has raised $29.5 million in five rounds from 13 investors, including a $23 million Series B investment in April 2014 led by Andreessen Horowitz and Kaiser Permanente Ventures. Duffy projects that Prevent will have some 20,000 subscribers in 2015, their greatest growth coming from employers and health plans.

For now, Prevent targets prediabetes, but is also adaptable to other chronic conditions, like high blood pressure, high blood fat (triglycerides) and obesity.

Omada Health may be a pioneer in the digital therapeutics space, but Duffy envisions a future in which the Prevent model will become mainstream. "I honestly think that 100 years from now, if you asked my great-grandkids what the science shows, it will be that the best recipe for patient engagement is peer-supported groups of people who have things in common working with some sort of digital facilitator, with shared goals on a timeline. I think that's the recipe and I don't think that's ever going to change. Innovators will come up with better ways to make that recipe more and more refined, but the basics won't change."

WELLDOC: A MOBILE PRESCRIPTION THERAPY

In 2013, WellDoc, a Baltimore-based startup, made history. Its flagship product, BlueStar, became the first mobile prescription therapy (MPT) approved by the FDA as a Class ll medical device for adults with Type 2 diabetes. Unlike typical consumer apps, MPTs like BlueStar require a prescription from a licensed medical professional and must follow the same privacy rules as providers. The FDA website notes, "These products are not like the simple health apps you can get for your phone or tablet. They can provide medical advice that regular apps aren't allowed to provide."

Simply put, BlueStar is not your average disease management app. According to Anand Iyer, WellDoc's chief data officer, whom I quote at the beginning of this chapter, an MPT is "the convergence of mobile technology, clinical behavioral science and validated clinical outcomes that create a new world healthcare solution to support patients in their daily self-care and give their healthcare provider additional data and insights to support clinical decisions."

The BlueStar system is built on automated clinical coaching and behavioral algorithms driven by real-time patient data. Instead of following the typical protocol of having users just test their blood sugar during the day, BlueStar software guides each patient in learning the *optimal* time to test his or her sugar—the multi-point profile. In this way, a patient gets a more accurate picture of how blood sugar may fluctuate throughout the day and what's driving those fluctuations. BlueStar not only helps people regulate their blood sugar and medication with more precision, but also provides in-the-moment automated coaching and tips.

According to Iyer, "The goal is to guide the patients on how to better manage their diabetes and stay within the recommended parameters set by their physician and the published guidelines. Yes, it's about behavior modification for the patient, but it's also about using data to drive clinical insights for the provider and improve outcomes." Although WellDoc has focused on Type 2 diabetes, the platform can be adapted for different chronic illnesses.

WellDoc was founded in 2005 by Suzanne Sysko Clough, MD, an endocrinologist, and her brother Ryan Sysko. That same year, Iyer, then director of the Wireless Industry Group at PRTM Management Consultants, met Clough at a Qualcomm event in New York City. They hit it off. During several conversations over the next several days, Clough expressed her frustration over the fact that in between office visits her diabetic patients retained very little of the information she provided on how to manage their disease. As Iyer recalls it, "She described how her patients struggled when they left her office. She said, 'I try my best, but when I see them again in three months, it's like I taught them a foreign language and they didn't get to practice it.'" Iyer served as a consultant to WellDoc until he joined the company full-time in December 2007.

Clough's observation resonated with Iyer, who had been diagnosed in 2002 with Type 2 diabetes. He knew first hand just how scary and complicated this disease could be for patients. As an expert in wireless technology, he was also intrigued by Clough's vision of building a platform that would use data and knowledge as a tool to change patient behavior.

Clough's vision was very radical thinking for 2005, two years before Steve Jobs had even *introduced* the iPhone. It was also well before the mass adoption of smartphones, during a time when even the most avid proponents of healthcare reform would not have dared to dream that the Affordable Care Act would be passed a few years later. As Iyer notes, "You can imagine the naysayers when we first said that we have a prototype solution model."

When the Apple App Store opened in 2008, WellDoc didn't just rush an app to market. Its mobile diabetes management platform underwent rigorous clinical trials to produce the kind of scientific data and evidence that the team could share with the FDA, as well as show to prospective clients, including pharmacy benefit managers (PBMs) and health plans seeking to improve patient adherence and outcomes.

Their studies yielded positive results. One randomized clinical trial, conducted with the University of Maryland and published in *Diabetes Care* in 2011, found "the combination of behavioral mobile coaching with blood glucose data, lifestyle behaviors and patient self-management data individually analyzed and presented with evidence-based guidelines to providers substantially reduced glycated hemoglobin levels over 1 year." The mean decline in glycated hemoglobin, or HbA1c, for the group using the WellDoc software was 1.9% versus 0.7% for people receiving usual care, resulting in a statistically significant difference of 1.2%. To put this in perspective, this is a significantly better result than the FDA requires for the approval of a new diabetes drug.

And if you think that the FDA was an impediment to their progress, Iyer says you'd be dead wrong. "Everybody accuses the FDA of slowing things down and getting in the way of innovation, when, in fact, we found it was quite the opposite. They wanted to understand. They asked us, 'Guys, please tell us what we all can do differently and we'll listen to each other.'"

Iyer says WellDoc's team did just that, explaining the potential of this new technology to key opinion leaders, members of Congress and FDA officials who were interested in championing change.

WellDoc achieved a major breakthrough in 2010, when the FDA granted the company 510(k) clearance to market its WellDoc DiabetesManager System to care providers and adult patients with Type 2 diabetes.

But the real challenge to this type of long-range project is finding investors who look beyond short-term gain. As Iyer points out, "Can you imagine a traditional Silicon Valley tech company going to a VC and saying: 'I want $20 million, or $10 million or even $5 million because I'm going to build a software app that I'm going to run through a clinical trial that may or may not work, that will probably take me two years, and if it does work, I'm then going to take it to the FDA, but there's a 50-50 chance that it may get shot down? Would you please fund that?'"

And yet, investors stepped forward. Merck Global Health Innovation Fund and Windham Venture Partners were Series A funders. One early investor, successful real estate developer and philanthropist Stewart Greenebaum, a patient of Clough's who was also struggling with diabetes, found that the WellDoc platform made it much simpler for him to control his blood sugar.

Says Iyer, "We continue to find investors who believe in demonstrating clinical evidence in digital health, even though it is a more unorthodox and even arduous path. WellDoc's goal is to continue to build products of very high clinical and economic value."

TWINE: A COLLABORATIVE CARE PLATFORM

"The patient is the most underutilized resource in healthcare," is the theme that has propelled physician John Moore's journey into connected health. His vision of the Digital Prescription began when he was a PhD candidate at the New Media Medicine Group at the MIT Media Lab. After leaving the Lab, he co-founded Twine Health with serial entrepreneur Frank Moss, PhD, former director of the Media Lab and the founder and current principal investigator for the New Media Medicine Group, and Scott Gilroy, a software developer also from the MIT Media Lab.

As I've mentioned previously, the Twine Collaborative Care Platform is a cloud-based platform, focusing on chronic ailments that require patient management, like hypertension, diabetes, heart failure, COPD and asthma. According to Moore, "Twine allows people to co-create a personalized care plan that serves as common ground for continuous collaboration with their care team." This is a team that includes their providers (physicians and/or nurse practitioners, for example) as well as family and friends. A human coach (nurse, pharmacist, health coach) is also an integral part of the Twine experience and shares a synchronized screen with the users.

To Moore, the differentiator for Twine is its core belief that patients must be involved in—and responsible for—their own healthcare. "If patients are not involved in that plan, if they haven't bought into it, they won't do it," he insists.

Once a patient enrolls in Twine, he sits down with his coach to discuss health goals and create a plan, which includes medication protocols and diet and exercise goals. From then on, the user inputs his blood pressure readings into his Twine account daily, as well as each time he takes his medication, eats and exercises. All the data appears on a real-time dashboard that, in addition to monitoring blood pressure and medication adherence, also displays how well the patient has been meeting his self-reported lifestyle goals. According to Moore, the presentation of data juxtaposed with this other vital information enables users to quickly contrast their actions with their outcomes. "It helps to highlight if there's a disconnect between what the person *thinks* he's doing, and what he's *actually* doing, and how it impacts his numbers," Moore says.

In addition to a coach, patients can choose to share their data with friends and family members.

Twine also enables patients to be active participants in all aspects of the decision-making process, including decisions traditionally left to doctors, like whether or not to change a medication or the dose. Moore explains, "We give users some of the algorithms that would be used by extenders (coaches) or by physicians. We found that they're extremely capable of understanding and asking questions like, 'Well, what would happen if I adjusted this medication up? What would happen if I adjusted it down?' Because, in those scenarios, it requires the input from the patient to do it. In turn, the physician or extender needs to know, 'What are the measurements? How are you feeling? Are you having any side effects? What's the variation like on a day to day basis?'"

In the Twine system, one coach can monitor a pool of 500 patients simultaneously; the platform enables coaches to quickly identify people who may need immediate attention based on the real-time data generated by the users. According to Moore, there are efficiencies to be gained by a provider who chooses to use this approach. "This technology platform doesn't have coaches calling people on the phone and leaving voicemails and bringing them into the office, all of those things that really drive down efficiency."

Even more importantly, Moore says, "The patient is so self-empowered, putting together so much more of the puzzle, that it leaves much less to be done by the coach or physician."

Peer-reviewed, published studies have shown that Twine can significantly reduce the annual cost of caring for a hypertensive patient (when compared to the conventional approach) by improving medication adherence, lowering blood pressure and reducing the number of follow-up visits. In one study published in 2014 in the *Journal of Clinical Outcomes Management* (*JCOM*), 100% of patients reached a target blood pressure of 140/90 within 90 days. In standard care, only 30% of patients with uncontrolled blood pressure reach this target in a year. Not only that, Twine was less expensive to administer than conventional care. According to the publication, "Typically, interventions that produce downstream savings in healthcare require some upstream investment. An exciting aspect of this intervention is that it was significantly less costly, at $67.50 per patient, as compared with the standard of care, at $248 per patient per year."

As this study states, the promise of Twine, and other automated programs like it, is that "this more efficient and scalable model of care could allow a practice to care for a larger number of patients without compromising the experience for patients or clinician."

And that's exactly why investor Andy Palmer believes that Twine is a "no brainer" for Accountable Care Organizations and other providers and payers looking at both the bottom line and quality of care. He says, "The cost of Twine is trivial, it's nothing. It's these kinds of solutions that are required in order to radically reduce the cost of providing care while, at the same time, creating dramatically better outcomes."

Palmer also envisions a time when consumers who are concerned about their own health will subscribe to a service like Twine on their own. "It's really very simple. People will eventually understand that if you want to get your blood pressure under control, you will use a system like Twine," he asserts.

In our work at Partners Connected Health, we have shown in a number of instances (detailed elsewhere in this book) that:

- An automated texting program can improve diabetes as well as or better than standard oral pharmacologic therapies.
- For teenagers with asthma, being part of a Facebook group can improve their outcomes as well as an inhaler.
- Patients on home monitoring for hypertension have a significant drop in blood pressure independent of what medications they are on.

These are all examples of the concept of Digital Rx.

Why is this important? It takes 20 years on average to bring a new drug to market and at great cost. There is also incremental cost in manufacturing drugs and keeping them in the supply chain. It takes a comparatively short time to build and verify the utility of a mobile app. Once the utility is verified, scale comes easily.

The idea that software can compete with chemical therapeutics opens up all kinds of business opportunities:

- As we turn our attention, societally, to battling chronic, lifestyle-related illnesses, we are relearning the power of behavioral health, motivation and engagement.
- We've ushered in the era of the digital therapeutic.

- The three companies featured in this chapter serve as examples of how the concept of digital therapeutics can thrive in the marketplace.
- There are now many well-documented instances of where digital solutions achieve outcomes equivalent or better than conventional chemical therapeutics.
- The business opportunity lies in how easy it is to develop, test, modify and prove utility for software and how easy it is to scale once developed.

12

The Privacy Trade-Offs

"I think that the minimum commitment for a developer is to be honest with people about what you're doing. Some people can then choose to leave the service that you're offering based on their privacy sensitivities; some may decide to stay. That decision will depend on whether or not they believe using the product is valuable enough to make them willing to accept the trade-offs."

—Deven McGraw, deputy director for Health
Information Privacy, U.S. Department of Health &
Human Services, Office for Civil Rights

When the topic of privacy makes headlines, it's usually spun in a negative context. The cyber world is most often presented as a place where consumers are continually duped and exploited, their data leaked or stolen and even seemingly well-meaning gestures on the part of companies are seen in sinister overtones. Here are a few illustrations of what I mean:

- A *New York Times* headline in June 2015 proclaimed, "Sharing Data, but Not Happily." Apple's Tim Cook, quoted in the article, cautioned, "You might like these so-called free services. But we don't think that they're worth having your email or your search history or now even your family photos data-mined and sold off for God knows what advertising purposes."

- "Weighing Privacy Vs. Rewards Of Letting Insurers Track Your Fitness," was the title of NPR's piece on John Hancock's innovative move in spring 2015 to offer lower life insurance premiums and rewards points to people willing to wear activity trackers and report their data to the insurance company. "This is essentially a medical surveillance system," warned Jamie Court of Consumer Watchdog, as quoted by NPR. "This may look like a carrot to lure new customers, but it's ultimately a stick."

- The recent cyber attacks on health insurers Anthem and Premera, among others, spawned a slew of stories like the one that appeared on April 14, 2015, in *USA Today*, entitled "Health Data Breaches Sow Confusion, Frustration." In the article, Ann Patterson, senior vice president and program director for the Medical Identity Fraud Alliance, an industry group, noted that medical identity theft poses a more serious threat to consumers than credit card fraud. She warned, "You really can't change your birth date. So when that kind of information is out there, the type of fraud that is perpetrated in the health care sense involves your well being, your life."

Is it any wonder that some consumers may be worried about data sharing?

Certainly, I understand that no one wants to feel spied on and vulnerable, and that data breaches are worrisome to all involved. Having said this, I wonder why we never see the other side of the story, particularly from the healthcare perspective. By that I mean, we don't talk about the value that can be created by all of this data and that can ultimately lead to improved health and improved care. We need to have this discussion, because if consumers don't understand the different sides of this complex story, there may be a push for more regulation, when in fact what's needed is more information and choice.

For a long time, despite the concerns of privacy advocates, this issue remained under the radar. It was brought to the forefront in the fall of 2015 when Facebook used its newsfeed to conduct a research study—unbeknownst to its members—evaluating how different types of posts may impact mood. When Facebook members found out that they had been experimented on without their knowledge, they were furious. You can argue that no one was hurt by the experiment, but it made more people wary of Facebook and raised red flags about how social media sites can use data.

Given the tendency of Facebook users to post all kinds of personal information online, this rebellion probably came as a surprise to Facebook's management. Granted, Facebook has a reputation for acting first and asking for forgiveness later—in terms of privacy, it continually pushes the envelope. This approach won't work for health.

First, the purveyors of health devices and consumer websites need to be even more cognizant of maintaining a bond built on trust. Individuals who purchase health services and health tracking devices need to feel that they are in a safe and comfortable environment. Second, if we're asking consumers to give up some of their privacy, we need to answer the age-old question, "What's in it for me?"

LEARNING FROM AN OLD MODEL

The real story is that privacy in the twenty-first century is about trade-offs—the exchange of personal data for some form of reward. Smart program designers need to make these trade-offs palatable to consumers and the potential rewards need to be so compelling that consumers understand what they are gaining in return. And, ultimately, it must be voluntary.

Once again, we can look to the advertising industry to provide a viable new model for health. The concept of providing consumers with something free to capture their attention in exchange for showing them advertising is not new. Most folks alive today grew up with the model where television content was free to the viewer, but for every 20 minutes of programming there was 10 minutes of advertising. Advertisers used very basic tools (such as surveys done by the Nielsen company) to target these ads. For instance, Ford and Coors can safely bet that folks who watch professional football will be more likely to be interested in purchasing a pickup truck or a Coors Light than those watching a figure skating competition. This level of targeting does not seem invasive to anyone.

Likewise, I get an envelope of coupons in the mail from time to time from local businesses—this type of advertising is segmented by zip code. I'm sure you can think of other examples that seem innocuous enough. Also, it's worth pointing out that when done right, this kind of targeting is even useful to the consumer. Isn't having a coupon for the new restaurant in the neighborhood useful if I was going to try it anyway? And, after collecting those coupons for a month or two, why shouldn't the restaurant in question decide in what zip codes to further target its advertising.

Enter the concept of trade-offs. The advertising industry is built on asking you to trade something (at a minimum a bit of your attention) for something else you perceive to be discounted or free. It has never been free. The currency, rather than dollars, is your attention or your personal information.

We now find the ad industry undergoing a transformation—advertisers are moving away from conventional media to online and mobile outlets. Why? New forms of media have access to more personal information based on tracking consumer buying habits, social media activity and other behaviors. Companies, like conventional newspapers and broadcasters, that are relying on the old way of doing business are losing out. In August 2015, for five days in a row, the Dow Jones Industrial Average slipped due to declines in ad revenues to video providers such as Viacom. Online advertisers can sell ads for three to seven times as much if they are targeted. Not surprisingly, this targeting has become the holy grail of Google, Facebook, Twitter and others.

In its simplest form, the tension around privacy is that advertisers want to extract more value from you for the same amount of that currency we talked about—your attention. Vacuuming up your digital bread crumbs and turning them into a highly personalized, targeted stream of ads is very lucrative. It is in the business interest of the companies who do this to be anything from vague to secretive about how they get this done, because you might demand more for your personal data if you know it's worth so much. Renowned computer scientist, philosopher, musician, and social critic Jaron Lanier beautifully lays out this concept in his 2013 book, *Who Owns the Future?*, in which he suggests that people should be able to *sell* their personal data on an open market. Fascinating.

OK, but how is this relevant to health? There are some definite parallels. The first one to come to mind is the insurance industry. Actuaries have been segmenting us for decades, giving insurers a sense of our risk of incurring costs and therefore the premium cost we should bear. The Ford truck ad on Monday Night Football doesn't feel invasive because it is so poorly targeted it doesn't enter your consciousness. It's directed to all men who watch football and buy cars. In contrast, the ubiquitous life-insurance physical may feel more invasive because the very purpose of the exam is to collect biometric data about *you*. More and more companies are doing the same—they're asking employees to undergo biometric screenings to more carefully segment their risk from an insurance perspective.

I think you can see where this is headed. By the end of 2015, 20 million U.S. homes will be "smart," in other words, laden with sensors connecting everything from the doorbell to the refrigerator to the Internet. In just the second quarter of 2015, Fitbit sold 4.5 million activity trackers! Soon, these personal health devices, like your Withings blood pressure cuff, your Proteus digital health medication adherence data, and more, will all be available in the cloud. It's a safe bet that those organizations that have bottom lines impacted by the health behaviors of their employees or customers will be dying to get such data into their predictive analytics programs to finely segment your risk and thus predict your cost and premiums.

The privacy conundrum hinges on the fear that somehow if "they" know this information about me, they will treat me unfairly in the insurance game. The memory of health insurers not covering preexisting conditions is still fresh, especially among those who were denied coverage. It may also be true that we are a bit more concerned about protecting our health data than, say, our online shopping habits, and for good reason. If we return to the concept of trade-offs, then, will the insurer (or the provider organization at risk) give you fair value for this data? And most importantly, will they take on the responsibility of protecting it? Or will they go the way of Facebook and try to pull the wool over your eyes?

WHAT CONSUMERS STAND TO GAIN

Consumers stand to gain a great deal from sharing their data, a fact that is often overlooked in privacy discussions. The same information that could help drive healthcare costs down can be used to create highly individualized programs that will help people stay healthier and happier. I've talked about how data can be used in a more positive light throughout this book, but what's highly interesting to me is that the message is not getting out to consumers.

Clearly there is an argument to be made that allowing a third party to monitor your data could work to your advantage, if it results in the early detection—or even prevention—of common physical and mental health problems. For example, just imagine if you wore an activity tracker and agreed to give your health insurer or provider access to your data in exchange for a lower premium (a classic trade-off). And let's suppose that "they"—the ones monitoring your data—detect a marked change in activity and sleep patterns over a four-week period. You then get a text or a call asking if anything is wrong, and that makes you realize that you've been working nonstop, have not been taking your usual walks every day and have been feeling very stressed out. Your insurer or provider then helps you get back on track by regularly sending you customized daily texts, reminding you to move, watch your alcohol intake and get enough sleep. Periodically, you get suggestions for how to relieve stress and even some discount coupons for a massage at your local spa.

Or let's suppose you have a history of depression. What if your healthcare management team asks if you would be willing to download an app that tracks your cell phone activity—and share that data with them—because it's been shown that this data can accurately predict depression before you may even be aware of a problem.

It is at this point in the dialogue when I hear cries of privacy invasion and comments like, "Gee, that sounds kind of creepy; they're spying on me." In reality, we allow marketers to do similar things behind our backs (like monitor our purchases or the websites we visit) because we understand we're getting something in exchange, like discount coupons, or offers only available to loyal customers.

Take the examples of Google Search and Google Maps. When I tap in one or two characters in the search bar, the vast majority of the time Google correctly guesses what I want to search for and allows me to autofill my intended topic. I like this. It's convenient for me and makes me want to use Google more. When I use Google Maps as a navigation system, it knows what destination I'm searching for in the same way, estimates travel time and helps me pick out the best route, all for *free*. Once again, this makes me want to use this product more. In both cases, Google can achieve these conveniences by collecting lots of private information about me (and others). *To me, this great product experience is worth the trade-off.* We can do the same with health data collection and health messaging.

The ability to share data with friends and colleagues via Facebook or Twitter is another tool that has been shown to help motivate some people to stay on track with their health and wellness goals. And the value of sharing data extends beyond social purposes: Some patient groups are banding together to offer their data to medical researchers, or are even conducting their own form of research. These kinds of activities may ultimately lead to new methods of treating and possibly even curing some diseases. Making it too difficult to exchange this kind of information could actually be harmful.

There's no question, the rights of individuals need to be protected—consumers must be in control of their own data and there must be complete transparency in terms of how it's being used. Consumers also need to feel safe. Recent breaches of patient data have deepened both patient and physician concerns about privacy. Individuals must feel that their personal health data is secure, presenting another big opportunity for businesses to step in and create solutions to address these problems.

Of course, breaches may occur, but, remember, they also happened in the analog era. In fact, at Partners HealthCare, a significant security breach occurred when an employee mistakenly left a printout of patient data on a subway car! Consumers need to understand this topic better, which means business needs to do a better job explaining it. There may come a time, however, when you'll be asked to decide if your requirement to keep information protected is worth a price. For example, are you willing to pay a higher insurance premium in exchange for remaining anonymous? These will be challenging conversations from a societal, legal and regulatory perspective.

HONESTY BUILDS TRUST

When I have legal questions about privacy issues, I turn to Deven McGraw, a former partner in the healthcare practice at Manatt, Phelps & Phillips, and now deputy director for Health Information Privacy for the U.S. Health & Human Services (HHS) Office for Civil Rights (OCR). I quoted her at the start of this chapter. What I like is her balanced view on the topic. Although she is a strong privacy advocate, Deven has represented a number of health startups and has recognized the mutual benefit of connected health for both consumers and businesses. If more companies followed her advice, we'd be further along in gaining the trust of the public.

As McGraw notes, part of the problem is that many businesses have either inadvertently or deliberately made it a point to keep consumers out of this discussion. They offer consumers complicated and nearly unreadable privacy policies that dictate the terms of the arrangement. She points out, "The problem is that we've got study after study after study that shows that these privacy policies either, in some cases, are nonexistent or hard to find or are very hard to read and don't always disclose what is actually going on with the app."

What exactly are the legal obligations of people who sell consumer health devices and apps? It's complicated. All medical data collected by providers or used in a medical record falls under the Health Insurance Portability and Accountability Act (HIPAA) Privacy Rule. According to the Health & Human Services website, the HIPAA Privacy Rule "provides federal protections for individually identifiable health information held by covered entities and their business associates and gives patients an array of rights with respect to that information. At the same time, the Privacy Rule is balanced so that it permits the disclosure of health information needed for patient care and other important purposes."

But once devices are in the hands of consumers, or data is posted outside of EMRs, the rules may change. To clarify, any medical data derived from a medical device—collected from a blood pressure cuff or glucometer, for example—that goes into a patient's medical record or is handled by a provider or payer, must be HIPAA compliant. But if a patient tweets the same data to a friend, posts it on Facebook, or stores it on a health app or smartphone, it is no longer under the same stringent regulations.

Apps and devices that collect data for nonmedical purposes, like activity trackers, weight scales, online food diaries, for example, are not subject to Federal privacy laws, but most of the companies creating these products provide their own privacy policies.

The state of California is the one exception to the rule about apps and devices: In 2013, California enacted amendments to its privacy law, the Confidentiality of Medical Information Act, to extend it to *any* hardware or software that collects medical information on behalf of a consumer. So if you sell your wares in California, you need to follow these stricter rules or risk being fined. (For more information on the California law, I refer you to an article written in September 2014, by McGraw and Susan Ingargiola, entitled "Confidentiality of Health Information in PHRs and Mobile Health Apps in California," which was published in *California Healthline*.)

CONSUMERS *DO* CARE

Although there is a common belief that the popularity of social networks has desensitized people—especially the young—to privacy concerns, that may not be entirely true. According to a study from the Annenberg School for Communication at the University of Pennsylvania, which the *New York Times* covered on June 6, 2015, 91% of respondents disagreed with the statement, "If companies give me a discount, it is a fair exchange for them to collect information about me without my knowing it." And 65% agreed with the statement, "I've come to accept that I have little control over what marketers can learn about me online." *If consumers feel that you're operating behind their backs, there will ultimately be a backlash.*

McGraw predicts that if companies don't start putting forth straightforward and clear privacy policies, the government will step in. "I think without a doubt that the Federal Trade Commission is going to crack down on companies that don't have a policy at all, and they'll also do it if that policy is very hard to find or hard to read and not completely clear with respect to how they use data," she says. And she goes on: "As we know, the Federal Trade Commission has already cracked down on companies for those reasons and if companies continue to be elusive with people about this, they will certainly hear from the FTC. In addition, states like California are thinking that the Feds are not doing enough in the space and are starting to enforce their own regulations."

In summary, privacy is not a very complicated issue—in fact, it's pretty straightforward. Below are two, in my opinion, pretty obvious tips on how to better work with consumers in an open, transparent way, which will ultimately work for everyone.

- Anyone who is in the health space, whether you're a payer, a provider or an entrepreneur who is developing devices or programs for consumers, needs to be very forthcoming about data collection and privacy policies. Make sure that the information you provide consumers is written in simple, easy to understand, nonlegalese.

- There's no such thing as a free app. And this is something that needs to be explained to consumers. If you're offering a free service, the usual business model is to sell advertising and often to sell data—including subscriber lists—to marketers. In most cases, if you were unable to create revenue this way, you would have to charge users a fee. This is not complicated; I believe users will understand. Some consumers may prefer a free service in which they give up some privacy; others will want a fee-based service that totally preserves their privacy. It should be the consumer's choice.

Afterword

What's Next?

Making predictions about the future is a risky business, yet that's exactly what we have to do to avoid being blindsided by it. No one can say with certainty what the healthcare system will look like in the next decade or so, but I can say with some degree of confidence that there are clear trends as to where we are headed.

I'm proud to say that Partners Connected Health has a solid track record in choosing to embark on projects that, in retrospect, make us seem prescient: Videoconferencing in the 1990s, second opinions via the Internet in 2001, congestive heart failure telemonitoring in 2003, texting as a tool for health messaging in 2008, and integrating patient-generated data into electronic medical records in 2012 are but a few examples. In each case, what was often initially dismissed by conventional medicine as impossible, too risky or simply "not the way things are done" eventually found its way into the mainstream.

I don't think that it diminishes the value of our accomplishments to admit that, with nearly all of these projects, we felt confident we knew how the future would play out. We believed that the world would turn out as we envisioned. Although we were virtually always correct on the big picture, we were often off—quite off—on some of the details.

For example, in 2003 we were working on a project using mobile phones as the gateway device for gathering and transmitting patient-generated data from the home. But we didn't envision the smartphone and how the user interface popularized by Apple would change the utility of mobile phones and lead to HealthKit, ResearchKit and so on. As we've come to realize, trying to predict the future is like looking into a room through an old-fashioned keyhole. You can see some features of the furniture and get a glimpse of the wall color, but you can't get the full perspective until you open the door and take in the whole scene.

There's a lesson to be learned from this. It makes sense to follow your instincts when working on the future, and it is critical to maintain flexibility in your thinking. You must also protect your innovation so that someone else doesn't come into the picture, snag your innovation, mainstream it and capture all of the credit.

So with the caveat that the future will most definitely hold some big surprises, those of you working to develop health technologies and innovations that will change care delivery know that you have an opportunity to literally create the future in a way that benefits mankind in the process.

To end this book, I've chosen to highlight six trends that are inevitable and to point out the connected health implications of each.

TREND 1: INCREASED LONGEVITY = INCREASED CHRONIC ILLNESS

It is a certainty that as time goes on we'll live longer, have more chronic illness and use more healthcare resources. As I've said throughout this book, budget-busting diseases such as hypertension, diabetes and congestive heart failure are all on the rise. Likewise, all of the "pre's"—*pre*diabetes, *pre*hypertension and the *pre*cursor of nearly all chronic disease, obesity—are increasing at an even faster rate. We can also count on the physician/nursing education process to fail to graduate proportionately more healthcare providers. Thus the current grumblings from the provider sector regarding being overworked, stressed and burdened with administrative details will only amplify. They (doctors, nurses, nurse practitioners and physician assistants) will readily perceive that they are in short supply. They will either leave the profession, creating even more perceived shortages, or demand more for their efforts. This is basic supply and demand. This phenomenon will also make providers even more vulnerable to disruption than they are today. *Think of CVS and Walgreens, whose innovations* *are described earlier in this book. They will continue to provide convenient, customer-friendly medical services, at first in the realm of urgent care, but eventually taking on more and more of what we think of as primary care.*

TREND 2: THE NETWORKING OF CARE AND THE CHALLENGE FOR THE HOSPITAL

We find ourselves in the middle of a 50- to 75-year journey that will result in a mostly virtual healthcare system. It is inevitable. When I was a child in the 1960s, the hospital *was* the information system. Now, like so many other services, healthcare delivery is becoming decentralized. In another 20 to 30 years, the hospital will be in one of two states. Either it will be a place for highly specialized, acute care (true emergencies, ICU and complicated surgeries) or it will reimagine itself as a wellness center and provide a value-added environment for the consumer/patient. The hospital of the future may enable its "customer" to get one-stop shopping for everything from a massage to a cardiac bypass.

The hospital faces the biggest challenge of all participants in the healthcare value chain. With significant investment in fixed assets, it is very difficult for hospital administrators to take any risk as they see this future unfold. *There is a business opportunity in the services/consulting realm to help hospital administrators manage this difficult transition.*

TREND 3: MOVING FROM VOLUME TO VALUE... NOT SO CLEAR

Will the movement toward value-based contracting for physicians and hospitals stick? Will this be the answer to the challenge of bending the cost curve? This is a prediction I'm less certain of. On the one hand, holding doctors and hospitals accountable for the quality and efficiency of the care they provide makes sense. We generate a significant portion of healthcare costs with the prescription pen and/or by ordering tests. Medicare, the biggest payer, is throwing its weight behind this solution. Perhaps if we work at it long enough, it will succeed. It may require a generation change though: The physicians who are used to the old way of doing business will need to move on/retire in order to make way for new, more open-minded practitioners.

Physicians are in a complicated position. We control revenue flow in the old system and enjoy everyone's respect. In the value-based world, we're more like tradesmen and have much less authority. Which would you choose? Experiments with value-based contracts (otherwise known as Accountable Care) have been mixed, with more scenarios where providers lost money than made money.

All of this simply makes it even more challenging for those selling care coordination and care efficiency services. We often counsel those folks to target "the one who is at risk." This used to be the health plan. Nowadays, it can be a health plan or a healthcare provider (ACO). Providers and plans look at the world differently, so they require different sales strategies. *A flexible sales strategy is advised for at least the next five to 10 years, until we clarify who really is at risk.*

TREND 4: THE CONSUMERIZATION OF HEALTHCARE IS A FACT OF LIFE

Another variable involves the consumerization of health cost decision making. It seems the trend is to shift more costs and decision making to individuals via high-deductible health plans, health savings accounts and health insurance exchanges. As a result, consumers will become increasingly cost conscious and start comparing services on price. No one who provides a service for a living wants that, because competing on price means relentless attention to costs. There's no room for premium services at premium pricing. Healthcare providers are not thought of as being committed to consumer/patient service. That's why the choice between competing on price and competing on service will be difficult for them. Providers that can get ahead of the curve on these two choices will reap benefits and those businesses that help them will as well.

We often talk about how healthcare is one of the few remaining services on the planet where you have to travel to a physical location and sit in the same room as the service provider to be served. People are fond of saying "consumers will expect more." And indeed they will. Many also predict that consumers, because of their experience with the "always on, always available" mobile marketplace—think of Airbnb and Uber—will demand that healthcare services be delivered in the same way. This is less certain. We've done a good job, over centuries, to convince people they must see their doctor (in person) to get quality healthcare.

The question is whether there will be enough consumer choice to enable market forces to work. If Walgreens, UnitedHealthcare and others succeed in offering competitive, consumer-friendly services at a lower price, then consumers will have choices and providers will have to respond. If providers manage to maintain their monopoly on providing care, little will change. *My advice to businesses is not to make a choice just yet, but to remain vigilant and flexible on this variable.*

TREND 5: CONNECTED HEALTH TECHNOLOGIES ARE HERE TO STAY. PERIOD.

What about technology and what role will it play? The Internet of Healthy Things is real and has longevity. The power of connecting previously inanimate objects, harnessing their data and applying machine-learning algorithms to improve products is proven in many areas. With our challenges of high demand and limited supply, this type of innovation will be hard to resist.

There are already examples of companies (Oscar, the New York City–based health insurance company, to name one) giving away smart activity trackers to members in order to gain access to day-to-day data in a number of prized demographics. As I detailed in Chapter 12, there will be a tug of war between those who want to harness all of the minutia and detail about each of us in order to customize service offerings and those who view that as an invasion of privacy. This will come to a head when some organization asks customers to make a decision between preserving privacy and paying a premium for a service delivered with that extra layer of privacy. In the meantime, there will be all kinds of room for innovation in this space, such as improved strategies for gathering and normalizing relevant patient-generated data, the analytics challenges around processing it all and the ability to use the insights gained to engage consumers in sustained, healthy behavior change.

What about virtual visits? They are all the rage right now, especially with forward-thinking providers. You can bet that virtual visits will be a mainstream part of healthcare delivery in the very near future. The technology is ubiquitous and easy to use, health plans are starting to reimburse for these visits and patients love the convenience. Virtual visits offer a viable alternative for many of those instances where doctors used to schedule a brief, targeted follow-up visit.

But at some point providers will figure out that video visits aren't more efficient. Because a virtual video visit binds two people in real time, the provider cannot provide one-to-many service. Yes, virtual visits can be delivered with reduced overhead costs. And the convenience factor for patients has real value. There's no question that our modern healthcare delivery system cares about patient loyalty and patient "leakage" and that virtual visits are one tool to accomplish this. At some point, though, we'll have to change to using as many one-to-many service models as possible.

Remote patient monitoring is not as far along on the adoption curve. However, you can safely assume that its adoption will grow. As ever more patients become facile with smartphones, apps and the like, the cost of remotely monitoring chronic conditions like hypertension and diabetes will go down. We've already shown that there is value in these patient-generated data, especially when they are combined with some sort of patient engagement overlay, such as nurse coaching or a social component, like sharing the data with your loved ones.

These programs are also convenient for patients, make them feel cared for and help them avoid high-cost events, such as office or emergency room visits and inpatient admissions. Some payers are beginning to create reimbursement strategies (led once again by Medicare). *While the virtual visit ship has sailed and the vendor market is somewhat crowded, the remote monitoring space still has room for lots of innovation, particularly around creating programs that are easy to set up, easy to use for patients and inexpensive for providers to deliver.*

TREND 6: DIRECT-TO-CONSUMER SERVICES WILL EXPAND

Another technology-related trend is direct-to-consumer services, which are potentially very disruptive to conventional healthcare delivery. This story starts with retail clinics, now mostly based in pharmacies, but it has recently gone virtual with a variety of services being offered that allow consumers to access care delivery online, without a previous face-to-face relationship. A few examples follow.

Some tasks that were handled by primary care providers are now conveniently handled by nurses in retail clinics. Because primary care is in such short supply, this has gone essentially unnoticed . . . so far. But once again, you see conventional hospitals and delivery systems launching urgent care clinics to compete. How long will it be before the retail clinic in your nearest pharmacy goes virtual?

As mentioned earlier, companies like CVS and Walgreens see primary care as a beachhead and chronic illness management as the hill to conquer beyond that. It only makes sense. While we as providers boast good relationships with our patients, the relationship patients have with their pharmacist is also quite strong. These companies plan to use technology to both make the urgent care setting virtual and to provide load balancing across sites (if the nurse practitioner at one site has a long wait, you can do a video consultation with the nurse practitioner at another site, if she is not busy at that moment).

Urgent care will become more and more convenient while institutionally based primary care will become more and more exclusive (logical if you perceive yourself to be in short supply). *If your company can be a supplier to the urgent care industry, you will likely be successful.*

In my field of dermatology, we have seen a number of websites spring up offering direct-to-consumer skin care services. Right now, they are targeting acne care, but with time you'll see that portfolio grow. You can measure the potential for disruption by the amount of attention organized dermatology is paying to this trend—it's generating a lot of discussion at national meetings.

Likewise, there are startups now offering to "Uber-ize" everything, including healthcare delivery. They will send a doctor to your house. This is interesting (and I suspect they will add a significant virtual care component to their service offering), but once again it's all disruptive to traditional healthcare delivery and particularly bread-and-butter stuff like immunizations, camp physicals, acne care and the like.

On a final note, the challenge of "selling health" to the consumer may prove to be the hardest task of all and one that requires the most thought and attention. Although it's true that devices like Fitbit, smart watches and smart clothing are "hot" commodities right now, whether they have legs remains to be seen. (We launched our own website, Wellocracy, to help consumers sort out how to evaluate trackers and choose the right one.)

This rapid growth is bound to slow down in the coming years, as all of the fitness/wellness/quantified-self apps and devices are chasing a relatively small market—the 5% to 10% of the population who are motivated to improve their health.

That's why I feel confident with this one last prediction: *If we want to truly transform the healthcare system, we need to entice the other 90% to get excited about self-tracking and, ultimately, become the managers of their own health.*

This is such an exciting time to be an innovator in healthcare. It's only going to get more turbulent, producing more opportunity for innovation.

Working in connected health for the past 20 years has been exhilarating for me (on most days, anyway). The rest of the world is catching up fast. We need as many entrepreneurs and innovators as possible to get involved. The demand for services continues to rise algorithmically and we already spend too much. The only way to fix it is to spread our healthcare provider resources across many more patients.

Technology has allowed that vision to flourish in other industries and we need to move that way in healthcare. But we have two added requirements: Patients must feel cared for and clinicians must be able to care for them. The broad goal of connected health is to achieve this one-to-many care model. We're well on the journey. I hope the lessons learned from this book will inspire you to get involved or, if you are already involved, I hope this book will help you avoid making some of the mistakes we've made along the way.

Select Bibliography

INTRODUCTION: MAKING THE CONNECTION

Agboola S, Jethwani K, Khateeb K, Moore S, Kvedar J. Heart failure remote monitoring: evidence from the retrospective evaluation of a real-world remote monitoring program. *J Med Internet Res.* 2015 Apr 22;17(4):e101. doi: 10.2196/jmir.4417. PubMed PMID: 25903278.

Broderick, Andrew. "Partners HealthCare: Connecting Heart Failure Patients to Providers Through Remote Monitoring." The Commonwealth Fund, January 2013.

Idriss SZ, Armstrong AW, Kvedar JC, Lio PA. Digital imaging in dermatology: attitudes, behaviors, and innovations. *Skin Res Technol.* 2009 Aug;15(3):376-7. doi: 10.1111/j.1600-0846.2008.00340.x. PubMed PMID: 19624436.

Pelletier A, McDermott L, Myint-U K, Kvedar JC. Text messaging to encourage prenatal care. *Female Patient* 2012;37(1):36-39.

Zan S, Agboola S, Moore SA, Parks KA, Kvedar JC, Jethwani K. Patient engagement with a mobile web-based telemonitoring system for heart failure self-management: a pilot study. *JMIR mHealth Uhealth* 2015 April 1;3(2):e33. doi: 10.2196/mhealth.3789. PubMed PMID: 25842282.

CHAPTER 2: SEEING AROUND CORNERS

"American Telemedicine Association Launches Program to Accredit Online Healthcare Services." News release, American Telemedicine Association, December 15, 2014.

Ask, JA. "mHealth Illustrates New Business Opportunities." *Forrester Research,* Cambridge, MA, February 4, 2014, updated February 24, 2014.

Burwell, SM. Setting value-based payment goals—HHS efforts to improve U.S. health care. *N Eng J Med.* 2015 Mar 5;372:10:897-9. doi: 10.1056/ NEJMp1500445. Epub 2015 Jan 26. PubMed PMID: 25622024.

Byrnes, Nanette. "Can Technology Fix Medicine?" *MIT Technology Review*, July 21, 2014.

Centers for Disease Control and Prevention. *National Diabetes Statistics Report: Estimates of Diabetes and Its Burden in the United States, 2014.* Atlanta, GA: US Department of Health and Human Services; 2014.

Coates SJ, Kvedar J, Granstein RD. Teledermatology: from historical perspective to emerging techniques of the modern era: part i: History, rationale, and current practice. *J Am Acad Dermatol.* 2015 Apr;72(4):563-574. doi: 10.1016/j.jaad.2014.07.061. PubMed PMID: 25773407.

————Teledermatology: from historical perspective to emerging techniques of the modern era: part ii: Emerging technologies in teledermatology, limitations and future directions. *J Am Acad Dermatol.* 2015 Apr;72(4):577-586. doi: 10.1016/j.jaad.2014.08.014. PubMed PMID: 25773408.

Consumer Intelligence Series: The Wearable Future. 2014 PricewaterhouseCoopers LLP.

Gandhi, Malay, and Teresa Wang. "Digital Funding 2015 Midyear Review." Rock Health, July 2015.

"The Internet of Things." *MIT Technology Review*, July/August 2014.

"Research and Markets: $173 Billion Wearable Technology Market Report 2015-2020. Analysis of 221 Companies Offering 132 Different Wearable Technology Products." *Business Wire*, February 12, 2015.

Smith, Aaron. U.S. Smartphone Use in 2015. Pew Research Center, April 1, 2015.

CHAPTER 3: THE BIG SHAKEUP

2014 Employer Health Benefits Survey. The Henry J. Kaiser Family Foundation, September 10, 2014.

Berwick, DM, Hackbarth, A. Eliminating waste in US healthcare. *JAMA.* 2012 April 11;307(14):1513-6. doi: 10.1001/jama.2012.362. Epub 2012 Mar 14. PubMed PMID: 22419800.

Chiu, Hewett. "Bringing Down Healthcare Costs: How can society promote affordability in the healthcare system?" *PolicyMatters Journal,* May 17, 2015.

"Chronic Care Management Services." Department of Health and Human Services, Medicare Learning Network. May 2015.

Dartmouth Atlas Project and PerryUndem Research & Communications. "The Revolving Door: A Report on U.S. Hospital Readmissions." Robert Wood Johnson Foundation, February 2013.

Friedman, Thomas L. *The World Is Flat: A Brief History of the Twenty-first Century.* New York: Farrar, Straus and Giroux, 2005.

"Health Care Costs: A Primer." The Henry J. Kaiser Family Foundation. May 1, 2012.

"Medicare's Delivery System Reform Initiatives Achieve Significant Savings and Quality Improvements - Off to a Strong Start." News release, HHS. gov, January 30, 2014.

Older Population as a Percentage of the Total Population: 1900 to 2050. Compiled by the U.S. Administration on Aging.

Physician Supply and Demand Through 2025: Key Findings. American Association of Medical Colleges, March 2015.

Rau, Jordan. "1,700 Hospitals Win Quality Bonuses From Medicare, But Most Will Never Collect." *Kaiser Health News,* January 22, 2015.

Unger, Laura, and Jayne O'Donnell. "Dilemma over deductibles: Costs crippling middle class." *USA Today,* Jan 1, 2015.

CHAPTER 4: THE HARDEST SELL

Agboola S, Havasy R, Myint-U K, Kvedar J, Jethwani K. The impact of using mobile-enabled devices on patient engagement in remote monitoring programs. *J Diabetes Sci Technol.* 2013 May 1;7(3):623-9. PubMed PMID: 23759394.

Bleich, SN, Bennett, WL, Gudzune, KA, Cooper, LA. Impact of physician BMI on obesity care and beliefs. *Obesity* (Silver Spring). 2012 May;20(5):999-1005. doi: 10.1038/oby.2011.402. Epub 2012 Jan 19. PubMed PMID: 22262162.

"Chronic Diseases: The Leading Causes of Death and Disability in the United States." National Center for Chronic Disease Prevention and Health Promotion, August 26, 2015.

Comstock, Jonah. "Report: 1.7B to Download Health Apps by 2017." *Mobihealthnews,* Mar 14, 2013.

"Consumer Wearable Market Demand Slowed Substantially From 2014 to Present After Hitting its Peak in January." News release and full report, *Argus Insights.*

Hale, Timothy M. "Is There Such a Thing as an Online Health Lifestyle? Examining the Relationship Between Social Status, Internet Access, and Health Behaviors." *Information, Communication & Society, Volume 16, Issue 4, 2013: 501-518.* doi:10.1080/1369118X.2013.777759.

Kuhnle GC, Tasevska N, Lentjes MA, Griffin JL, Sims MA, Richardson L, Aspinall SM, Mulligan AA, Luben RN, Khaw KT. Association between sucrose intake and risk of overweight and obesity in a prospective sub-cohort of the European Prospective Investigation into Cancer in Norfolk (EPIC-Norfolk). *Public Health Nutr.* 2015 Feb 23:1-10. [Epub ahead of print]. PubMed PMID: 25702697.

Ledger, Dan, and Daniel McCaffrey. "Inside Wearables: How the Science of Human Behavior Change Offers the Secret to Long-Term Engagement." Endeavour Partners LLC, January 2014.

Mobile Health Market Report 2013-2017. "The Commercialization of mHealth Applications (Volume 3)." Research2guidance, March, 2013.

Moore, Geoffrey A. *Crossing the Chasm: Marketing and Selling High Tech Products to Mainstream Customers.* New York: HarperCollins, 1991.

Pagoto, S, Schneider, K, Jokic, DeBiasse M, Mann D. Evidence-based strategies in weight-loss mobile apps. *Am J Prev Med. 2013 Nov;45(5):576-62. doi:* 10.1016/j.amepre.2013.04.025. PubMed PMID: 24139770.

Wansink, Brian. *Mindless Eating: Why We Eat More Than We Think.* New York: Bantam Dell, 2006.

CHAPTER 5: THE NEW WHITE COAT ANXIETY

"A Survey of America's Physicians: Practice Patterns and Perspectives." The Physicians Foundation, September 21, 2012.

Bernstein, Lenny. "How many patients should your doctor see each day?" *Washington Post.* May 22, 2014.

Jauhar, Sandeep. *Doctored: The Disillusionment of an American Physician.* New York: Farrar, Straus and Giroux, 2014.

Nass, Clifford, and Corina Yen. *The Man Who Lied to His Laptop: What We Can Learn About Ourselves from Our Machines.* New York: Current, Penguin Group USA, 2010.

Watson A, Bickmore T, Cange A, Kulshreshtha A, Kvedar J. An internet-based virtual coach to promote physical activity adherence in overweight adults: randomized controlled trial. *J Med Internet Res.* 2012 Jan 26;14(1):e1. doi: 10.2196/jmir.1629. PMID: 22281837.

CHAPTER 6: SOME HEALTHY DISRUPTION

Darkins, Adam. "Telehealth Services in the United States Department of Veterans Affairs (VA)." Veterans Health Administration, 2014.

Darkins, A, Kendall S, Edmonson, E, Young M, Stressel P. Reduced cost and mortality using home telehealth to promote self-management of complex chronic conditions: a retrospective matched cohort study of 4,999 veteran patients. *Telemed J E Health.* 2015 Jan;21(1):70-6. doi: 10.1089/tmj.2014.0067. Epub 2014 May 19. PubMed PMID: 24841071.

Jung, Alexandra. "Walgreens' strategic transformation." *Progressions 2012*: ey.com interview.

Mobile Technology Fact Sheet. Pew Research Center, 2014.

"VA Telehealth Services Served Over 690,000 Veterans In Fiscal Year 2014." News release, U.S. Department of Veterans Affairs, October 10, 2014.

CHAPTER 7: UP CLOSE AND HYPERPERSONAL

Jethwani K, Ling E, Mohammed M, Myint-U K, Pelletier A, Kvedar JC. Diabetes connect: an evaluation of patient adoption and engagement in a web-based remote glucose monitoring program. *J Diabetes Sci Technol.* 2012 Nov 1;6(6):1328-36. PubMed PMID: 23294777.

Prochaska, James O, John C Norcross, and Carlo C. DiClemente. *Changing for Good: A Revolutionary Six-Stage Program for Overcoming Bad Habits and Moving Your Life Positively Forward.* New York: HarperCollins, 2006.

"Teradata Global Survey: 90 Percent of Marketers Say Individualized Marketing is the Future." News release, Teradata, Jan 28, 2015.

Watson AJ, O'Rourke J, Jethwani K, Cami A, Stern TA, Kvedar JC, Chueh HC, Zai AH. Linking electronic health record-extracted psychosocial data in real-time to risk of readmission for heart failure. *Psychosomatics.* 2011 Jul-Aug;52(4):319-27. doi: 10.1016/j.psym.2011.02.007. PubMed PMID: 21777714.

Watson AJ, Singh K, Myint-U K, Grant RW, Jethwani K, Murachver E, Harris K, Lee TH, Kvedar JC. Evaluating a web-based self-management program for employees with hypertension and prehypertension: a randomized clinical trial. *Am Heart J.* 2012 Oct;164(4):625-31. doi: 10.1016/j.ahj.2012.06.013. PubMed PMID: 23067923.

CHAPTER 8: TRY A LITTLE DOPAMINE

Armstrong AW, Watson AJ, Makredes M, Frangos JE, Kimball AB, Kvedar JC. Text-message reminders to improve sunscreen use: a randomized, controlled trial using electronic monitoring. *Arch Dermatol.* 2009 Nov;145(11):1230-6. doi: 10.1001/archdermatol.2009.269. PubMed PMID: 19917951.

Bravata, DM, Smith-Spangler, C, Sundaram, V, Gienger AL, Lin N, Lewis R, Stave CD, Olkin I, Sirard JR. Using pedometers to increase physical activity and improve health: a systematic review. *JAMA*. 2007 Nov 21;298(19):2296-304. PubMed PMID:18029834.

Clayton, Russel B, Glenn Leshner, and Anthony Almond. "The Extended iSelf: The Impact of iPhone Separation on Cognition, Emotion and Physiology." Wiley Online Library, *Journal of Computer-Mediated Communication*. March 2015; 20(2):119-135.

Meeker, Mary, and Liang Wu. "Internet Trends D11 Conference." Kleiner Perkins Caufield Byers, May 2013.

Packard, Vance. *The Hidden Persuaders*. New York: Random House, 1957.

CHAPTER 9: MAKING DATA ACTIONABLE

Pettypiece, Shannon, and John Robertson. "Hospitals Are Mining Patients' Credit Card Data to Predict Who Will Get Sick." Bloomberg Business, July 3, 2014.

Singer, Natasha. "When a Health Plan Knows How You Shop." *New York Times*, June 28, 2014.

Zai AH, Ronquillo JG, Nieves R, Chueh HC, Kvedar JC, Jethwani K. Assessing hospital readmission risk factors in heart failure patients enrolled in a telemonitoring program. *Int J Telemed Appl*. 2013;2013:305819. doi: 10.1155/2013/305819. Epub 2013 Apr 27. PubMed PMID: 23710170.

CHAPTER 10: THE REINVENTION OF BIG PHARMA

Agboola SO, Ju W, Elfiky A, Kvedar JC, Jethwani K. The effect of technology-based interventions on pain, depression, and quality of life in patients with cancer: a systematic review of randomized controlled trials. *J Med*

Internet Res. 2015 Mar 13;17(3):e65. doi: 10.2196/jmir.4009. PubMed PMID: 25793945.

"CVS Caremark Medication Adherence Report Identifies Significant Opportunities for Health Care Cost-Savings Across All 50 U.S. States." News release, *PR Newswire*, June 27, 2013.

Langreth, Robert. "Cancer Docs Join Insurers in U.S. Drug-Cost Revolt." Bloomberg Business, May 7, 2014.

Tefferi, A, Kantarjian, H, Rajkuman, SV, Baker LH, Abkowitz JL, Adamson JW, Advani RH, Allison J, Antman KH, et al. In support of a patient-driven initiative and petition to lower the high price of cancer drugs. *Mayo Clin Proc.* 2015 Aug;90(8):996-1000. doi: 10.1016/j.mayocp.2015.06.001. Epub 2015 Jul 23. PubMed PMID: 26211600.

Walker, Joseph, and Brian Gormley. "Billion Dollar Health Startups." *Wall Street Journal*, February 26, 2015.

Whelan, Jeanne. "Doctors Object to High Cancer-Drug Prices." *Wall Street Journal*, July 23, 2015.

Yonker LM, Zan S, Scirica CV, Jethwani K, Kinane TB. "Friending" teens: systematic review of social media in adolescent and young adult health care. *J Med Internet Res.* 2015 Jan 5;17(1):e4. doi: /jmir.3692. PubMed PMID: 25560751.

CHAPTER 11: THE DIGITAL RX

"Achievements in Public Health, 1900-1999: Family Planning. Centers for Disease Control. *MMWR Weekly*, Dec 03, 1999 / (48)47;1073-1080.

Moore, JO. "A New Wave of Patient-Centered Care: Apprenticeship in the Management of Chronic Disease." *JCOM,* July 2012, Vol. 19, No. 7.

Moore, JO, Marshall MA, Judge, DC, Moss, FH, Gilroy, SJ, Crocker JB, Zusman, RM. "Technology-Supported Apprenticeship in the Management of Hypertension: A Randomized Controlled Trial." *JCOM,* March 2014, Vol. 21, No. 3.

Quinn, CC, Shardell, MD, Terrin, ML, Barr EA, Ballew SH, Gruber-Baldini AL. Cluster-randomized trial of a mobile phone personalized behavioral intervention for blood glucose control. *Diabetes Care.* 2011 Sep;34(9):1934-42. doi: 10.2337/dc11-0366. Epub 2011 Jul 25. PubMed PMID:21788632.

Sepah, SC, Jiang, L, Peters, AL. Long-term outcomes of a Web-based diabetes prevention program: 2-year results of a single-arm longitudinal study. *J Med Internet Res.* 2015 Apr 10;17(4):e92. doi: 10.2196/jmir.4052. PubMed PMID: 25863515.

————Translating the Diabetes Prevention Program into an Online Social Network. Validation against CDC Standards. *Diab Educ.* 2014 Apr 10;40(4):435-443. [Epub ahead of print], PubMEd PMID: 24723130.

CHAPTER 12: THE PRIVACY TRADE-OFFS

Armental, Maria. "Fitbit's Profit Rises as Sales Surge." *Wall Street Journal,* August 5, 2015.

Dwoskin, Elizabeth. "Ad-Blocking Software Will Cost the Ad Industry $22 Billion This Year." *Wall Street Journal,* August 10, 2015.

Farr, Christina. "Weighing Privacy Vs. Rewards Of Letting Insurers Track Your Fitness." NPR KQED *All Tech Considered,* April 9, 2015.

Hufford, Austen. "U.S. Stocks Drop on Media Meltdown." *Wall Street Journal,* August 6, 2015.

Lanier, Jaron. *Who Owns the Future?* New York: Simon & Schuster, 2013.

McGraw, Deven and Susan Ingargiola. "Confidentiality of Health Information in PHRs and Mobile Health Apps in California." *California Healthline.* September 22, 2014.

Ornstein, Charles. "Health Data Breaches Sow confusion, Frustration." *USA Today,* April 14, 2015.

Singer, Natasha. "Sharing Data, but Not Happily." *New York Times,* June 6, 2015.

at Walgreens, 77–84
Yorn feedback platform for, 103–105
consumerization of healthcare, 184–185
consumer-payer relationship, 27–28
Cook, Tim, 170–171
cookies, 114
Coors, 172
COPD
    co-morbidity of mental health and, 139
    Twine Collaborative Care Platform for, 165–168
coping skills, 95
Cornell University Food and Brand Lab, 51
corporate wellness programs, engagement rate of, 125
cost of healthcare. *See also* healthcare expenditures
    and adoption of health technologies, 41–42
    consumer awareness of, 31
    consumers' stake in, 32–33
    expected rise in, 24
    for hospital readmissions, 24
    for hypertension, 167
    as percent of GDP, 24
    with preventive medicine, 26
    quality of care and, 8
    splitting, between consumers and health system, 42
Coumadin, 152
Court, Jamie, 171
Crossing the Chasm (Geoffrey A. Moore), 46
culture of health, 44
current procedural terminology (CPT) reimbursement code, for chronic care
    management, 30–31
CVS, 78, 80, 147, 182–183, 187
CVS Health, 147

"Dilemma over Deductibles: Costs Crippling Middle Class," 31–32
direct data, 129
direct-to-consumer services, 186–188
disease burden, xxv
Doctored (Sandeep Jauhar), 61
doctors. *See* physicians
dopamine, 108
drones, 155–156
drug launches, 151–154
drugs. *See also* pharmaceutical industry; *specific drugs*
    biologics, 145
    biosimilars, 11, 144, 146
    generic, 36, 142, 146
    as loss leaders, 150
    medication adherence, 129, 144–146
    prices of, 144
    specialty pharmaceuticals, 142–144
DR Walk-In Medical Care, 83–84
DRX, 144
Duane Reade, 78, 83–84
Duffy, Sean, 159, 160, 162

ear infections, 42–43
early adopters, 46, 48–49
education
    inspiration vs., 52–53
    in medical school, 60, 62–63, 113
    in patient management, 69
    and provider shortages, 182
efficiencies, 23, 35
elderly home care, xxi
electronic medical (health) records (EMR), 13

generational diversity, 78, 83, 86, 88–89

generic drugs, 36, 142, 144, 146

genomics

  incorporated into EMRs, 101–102

  in predictive analytics, 131

gifts to physicians, 73

Gilead Sciences, 144

Gilroy, Scott, 166

Ginger.io, 126, 136–139

Glaser, John, xx

goals of patients, learning about, 111–113

Google, 11, 14, 46, 114, 117, 122, 136, 173, 176

Google Field Trip, 122

Google Health, 46

Google Maps, 176

Google Now, 14

Google Search, 176

Greenebaum, Stewart, 165

gym memberships, 45

Haiti, 155

Hale, Tim, 53–54, 96–97

Harvey, Noel G., 154–156

Havasy, Rob, 22

Hawthorne Effect, 119–120

health analytics. *See* data analytics

healthcare business

  business models for, 16, 62, 146–147, 150

  current changes in, xxv (*See also* changes in healthcare system)

  data analytics opportunities in, 131

  historical drivers of, 23

  market forces in, 10

high-deductible health plans, 9, 31–32
value-based reimbursement, 8
insurers, consumers' relationship with, 27–28
Intel, 11
Internet, availability of information on, 32
Internet of Healthy Things (IoHT), 5, 10, 185
    additional data sources in, 129
    and culture of health, 44
    ideal model for, 13–14
    participants in, 11–12
    and reinvention of healthcare system, 6
    and "stickiness" of technologies, 45
    tools for health through, 26 (*See also* Digital Rx)
Internet technologies, xvii. *See also individual technologies*
    for remote data transmission, 39–40
    for remote second opinions, xx
interoperability, 13
iPhone, controlling drones with, 156
iPhone separation, 106
ISPs, 36
ITM, 134
Iyer, Anand, 157, 163–165

James, Adrian, 159
Jantoven, 152
Jauhar, Sandeep, 57, 61–62
Jawbone Up, 15
Jethwani, Kamal, xxiv, 26, 39, 90
Johansson, Scarlett, 70
John Hancock, 171
Johns Hopkins Bloomberg School of Public Health, 53
Johns Hopkins Health System, 80
Jonze, Spike, 70

Nielsen, 172
nighthawk services, 37
Nike + FuelBand, 15
North Bridge Venture Partners, 134
Northwestern Memorial Hospital, 80
novel oral anticoagulants (NOACs), 152–154
NPR, 171
nudges, 114
nurses
  beliefs about face-to-face interactions among, 66–67, 69
  difficulty of change for, 60
  poor health behaviors among, 53
  primary care handled by, 187
  shortage of, 25

obesity, 20, 51
  effective treatments for, 158
  as epidemic, 158
  increase in, 182
  individual accountability for, 41
  and Prevent lifestyle intervention program, 159
objective data, 128
Omada Health, 159–162
Ommen, Steve R., 60, 64, 65
OM Signal, 11
one-to-many care model, 188
operant conditioning, 119
opioid addiction treatment, xxiii
Optum, 126, 134
Oracle, 126
O'Reilly, David, 149–150
Oscar, 185
Oto Home, 42–43

About the Authors

JOSEPH C. KVEDAR, MD

Joe Kvedar, vice president of Connected Health at Partners HealthCare in Boston, is creating a new model of healthcare delivery, developing innovative strategies to move care from the hospital or doctor's office into the day-to-day lives of patients. He is internationally recognized as a pioneer and visionary in the field of connected health.

CAROL COLMAN

Carol Colman is the co-author of more than two dozen books on health, wellness, antiaging and technology, including numerous *New York Times* and national bestsellers. She lives in Brooklyn, New York.

GINA CELLA

Gina Cella is the principal of Boston-based Cella Communications, a public relations firm representing leaders in the field of healthcare, promoting cutting-edge personal health technologies, provider organizations and biotech/pharma companies for the past two decades.

Made in the USA
Lexington, KY
14 October 2016

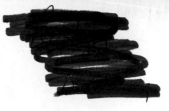

Nature's Nation

An Environmental History
of the United States

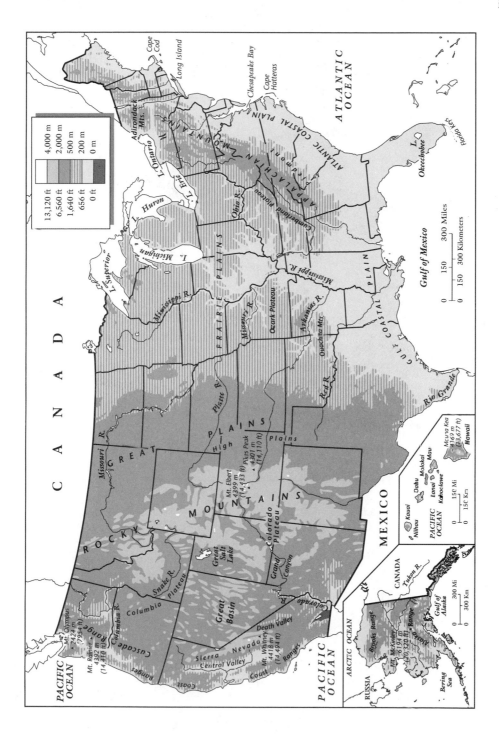

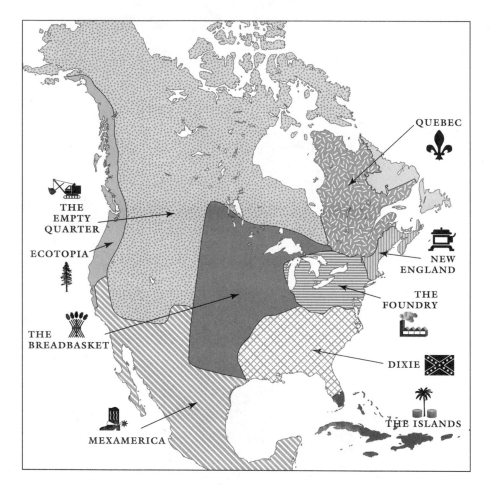

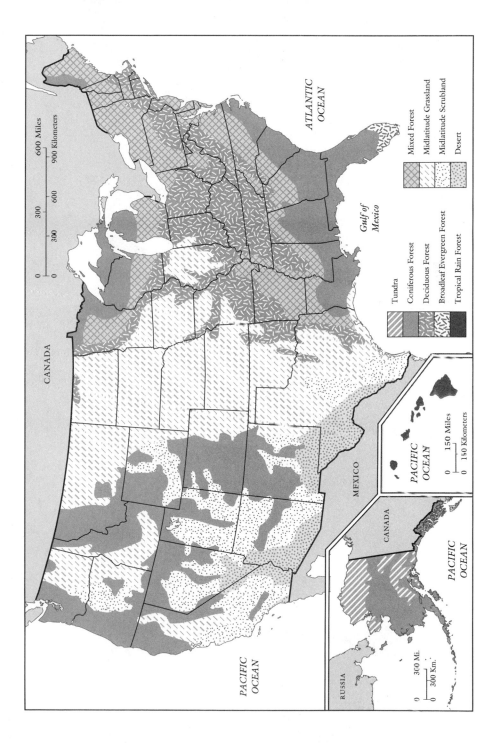

CANADA

ATLANTIC
OCEAN

Gulf of
Mexico

PACIFIC
OCEAN

MEXICO

PACIFIC
OCEAN

CANADA

RUSSIA

PACIFIC
OCEAN

600 Miles

900 Kilometers

0   300   600

0   300   600

0   150 Miles

0   150 Kilometers

0   300 Mi.

0   300 Km.

Tundra

Coniferous Forest

Deciduous Forest

Broadleaf Evergreen Forest

Tropical Rain Forest

Mixed Forest

Midlatitude Grassland

Midlatitude Scrubland

Desert